OUTSMARTING FEMALE FATIGUE

The 8 Energizing Strategies

for Lifelong Vitality

Debra Waterhouse, M.P.H., R.D.

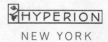

NEW YORK

The advice in this book is not intended for persons with chronic illnesses or other conditions that may be worsened by an unsupervised eating and/or exercise program. The recommendations are not intended to replace or conflict with advice given to you by your physician or other healthcare professional, and we recommend that you do consult with your physician. The author and publisher cannot be held responsible for any results arising from the use or application of the information in this book.

Except for those who have given permission to appear in this book, all names have been changed. In some cases, composite accounts have been created based on the author's professional experience.

Copyright © 2001 Debra Waterhouse

Library of Congress Cataloging-in-Publication Data

Waterhouse, Debra.
    Outsmarting female fatigue : 8 energizing strategies for lifelong vitality /
Debra Waterhouse.
        p.   cm.
    Includes bibliographical references.
    ISBN 0-7868-6538-5
    1. Women—Health and hygiene.   2. Fatigue—Prevention.   3. Vitality.
I. Title.

RA778 .W2189 2001
613'.04244—dc21

                                                      00–037029

Book design by Ruth Lee

FIRST EDITION

10 9 8 7 6 5 4 3 2 1

Outsmarting
Female Fatigue

For

TIMOTHY, MAX,
AND LUKE

*who always bring a smile to my face
and joy to my life*

Acknowledgments

It takes an immense amount of time and energy to write a book, a feat that would be exhausting were it not supported and encouraged by family, friends, and colleagues. I am grateful for having such a reenergizing support system in my life.

My sister, Lori Waterhouse Erwin, was once again my sturdy rock and guiding light. She tirelessly read every word again and again, giving me the direction and confidence I needed to keep going strong. After she gave her chapter-by-chapter approval, my editor, Leslie Wells, was ready and waiting, eager to offer her thoughtful input and enthusiastic feedback. And my agent, Sandy Dijkstra, whose unmatched vitality inspired this book, gave the final thumbs-up and the reassurance of a job well done. With these three spirited women by my side, my excitement for this project never faltered.

There is, however, a fourth special woman to acknowledge. Although Judith Riven was not directly involved in these pages, she was my editor for all my previous books and her keen guidance is forever ingrained. I found myself constantly asking, "Now how would Judith edit this paragraph?" Thank you, Judith, for permanently improving my writing skills.

I would also like to thank my dedicated reviewers, Dr. Dee Tivenan, M.F.C.C.; Stephanie Goulding, R.N.; Elizabeth Somer, M.A., R.D.; Joyce Gardiner Filatreau, Mary Pat Cedarleaf, Jeannette Highton Stansbury, and Stacey Marcus, for their valuable time and insight; my research assistants, Margaret Binkley and Katie Hawkins, for their fact-finding expertise; and my parents, Ray and Alina Waterhouse, who flew to California to take care of my new baby, Tyler (whose delivery came before I had a chance to deliver this manuscript), so I could make the final revisions on this book.

And last, I am forever indebted to the two special men in my life: my husband, Paul, for giving me his infinite patience and understanding, and my son, Tyler, for granting me an easy pregnancy and delivery. I wrote the majority of this book during his nine months of gestation, and he was kind enough to let them be free of morning sickness, insomnia, and fatigue.

Contents

WHY DO I FEEL
SO TIRED?

Chances are, this question has crossed your mind more than once today. You felt the wave of fatigue come crashing over your body, and the question hit you like a ton of bricks. But having neither the energy to figure out why nor the time to let yourself be tired, you grabbed another cup of coffee and forced yourself to move on to number 14 of 32 on today's to-do list.

If you could take the time to ponder this question, what would be your answer?

- **"I must not be organized enough."** Organized? With the amount you have to accomplish each day, even Martha Stewart couldn't keep her day planner organized by the minute, her desk clear of clutter, and her sock drawer lined up by color.

- **"Maybe I'm premenstrual."** While it's true that your fatigue level increases during PMS, you can't possibly be premenstrual all month long. You're actually in the middle of your cycle and should be at the peak of your energy, not the pit.

- **"I'm menopausal, so I'm supposed to be tired."** True again, but are you supposed to be *this* exhausted? Hot flashes can drain your energy, but you feel like you've been run over by a train.

- **"Maybe I have chronic fatigue syndrome."** Less than 1 percent of our fatigued population can be clinically diagnosed with chronic fatigue syndrome (or as it's called now, chronic fatigue immunodeficiency syndrome). For the rest of us, fatigue is not an illness. It's a chronic feeling of exhaustion caused by doing too much and resting too little.

- **"I must be fighting something."** Occasionally an intruder virus may be zapping your energy, but if it's not flu season, most likely the only thing you're fighting is your fatigue.

Daily, relentless fatigue is not due to viral invasion, an illness, organizational impairment, PMS, or menopause (although these can certainly intensify it). It's due to the reality that you're overworked, overstressed, overextended, and overwhelmed—and underrested, undernourished, underjoyed, and under a dark cloud. You *feel* tired all the time because you *are* tired all the time. And you're not alone.

The undisputed medical fact is: We're in a female energy crisis. At any given time of day or night, 80 percent of all women report fatigue. We drag ourselves out of bed, unrefreshed and anxious about the day, then rush through our day as we fall farther and farther behind schedule, and finally collapse in bed worn out and worried about tomorrow. Every woman I know personally and professionally makes some reference to how stressed, spent, worn-out, unhappy, or disconnected she feels. And those who don't come right out with a verbal declaration of their exhausted state of existence give more subtle signs. I can hear it in their labored speech or see it in their strained faces—the same dark circles and furrowed brow that are sometimes familiar from my own reflection.

Since "the mirror doesn't lie" is a widely accepted adage, let's use it. Go into the bathroom or take out your compact to view your face of fatigue. Do you look enthusiastically alive or dead tired? Even the best makeup job can't cover up fatigue. As you walked to the bathroom, did your steps come with ease or excruciating effort? When you're worn out, even a short journey can feel like a monumental feat. It's impossible to look, feel, or act vital when you are exhausted from stressful days, endless schedules, and/or sleepless nights. In the most basic sense, *energy is life*. It gives us the passion and enthusiasm to actively live. Without it, we passively go through the monotonous motions of life without truly living. It's no wonder that only 24 percent of us say that we have a good life, that more than 50 percent say that we feel sad more often than we feel happy, and that one in four women will experience major depression in their lifetimes. We feel depleted and defeated by our exhausting lives.

I have been helping women for almost twenty years by writing books, giving seminars, and providing counseling, and what saddens me most is that the majority of women I come across have resigned themselves to a life that lacks happiness, a heart that lacks passion, a soul that lacks spirit, eyes that lack sparkle, and a body that lacks nourishment. "That's just the way it is," they tell me. "I don't have the time, energy, or desire to be anything but exhausted. Maybe when the kids are out of the house, maybe when I'm twenty pounds thinner, maybe when my ship comes in, maybe when I win the lottery, maybe in my next life—things will be different and I'll have the time and energy to take care of myself."

Well, maybe your kids will live with you longer than you'd like, perhaps your body was meant to be a bit larger than that of an emaciated model, maybe your ship has sunk at sea, maybe you'll be one of the 999,999,999 who don't win the jackpot, perhaps this life is it. What then? Another ten or twenty or thirty years will go by and instead of wondering where your energy has gone, you'll wonder where your life has gone.

Needless to say, fatigue can be a real downer—in more ways than one. And despite the dismal topic, I want to give you some lightheartedness to lift your spirits and a positive approach to a negative subject. Every cloud has a silver lining—even the dark cloud of fatigue—and my goal is to help you find that silver lining, solve your personal fatigue crisis, and enjoy the journey to enhanced energy, balance, and peace. In other words, I want to help you give yourself the gift of living.

As with my other books written for women, these pages offer you a no-nonsense, biologically based program that works with the realities of your unique female body to unleash your inner energy and revitalize your life. If you are like many of my female friends, clients, and colleagues, you may be excited about the prospect of enhancing your energy and restoring your vitality. "Quick! Tell me now! What pills should I be taking? I've heard about ginseng, should I try it? How about B_{12} injections? Which energy bar is the best? Tell me what to do!"

My female circle knows me better than to ask about quick-fix megadoses, potions, drinks, injections, or bars. But you may not, so let me introduce you to the philosophies that guide everything I do.

- A woman's body is a miracle of engineering—from our premenstrual tension to our menopausal memory loss, from our food cravings to our mood swings, and from our expanding fat cells to our extreme fatigue—explanations exist for *everything* our bodies experience.

- Listen to and trust the wisdom of your female body—it's the expert in directing you down the path of health, vitality, and longevity.

- You are responsible for your own health and well-being—not me, a book, a pill, your partner, your homeopath, your doctor, or your therapist. **You have to take charge to recharge your energy**.

- There are no quick fixes or magical cures—if it sounds too good to be true, it probably is.

Historically, women's concerns have always been a magnet for the purveyors of unproven remedies and miracle cures—whether it be for PMS, menopause, aging, or weight loss. Just look to the diet industry as an example. For the past forty years, we have been presented with diet after diet, gimmick after gimmick, pill after pill, each leading us to believe that it is the magical solution to weight loss. Let's learn from the past. We have forty years of gimmicks, but we also have forty years of weight-loss research to prove that quick weight-loss diets don't keep their promises—but they certainly do keep piling the pounds on quickly. Since we started dieting in the 1960s, the average woman has added twenty-five pounds to the scale. We haven't lost any weight by dieting, but we have lost a lot of energy. Instead we've gained weight and increased our level of fatigue. Could there be a correlation here? As our dieting efforts and weights have climbed, our energy levels and vitality have plummeted. Maybe this is why they are called "crash diets."

It should come as no surprise that fatigue has recently tied with weight as a woman's primary concern—and the market is already flooded with products that claim to "banish fatigue" or "boost energy." Manufacturers are quick to respond to women's concerns, and their claims are convincing. What woman wouldn't be tempted by the promise of youthful energy, sustained stamina, everlasting vitality—and sometimes permanent weight loss at the same time? But promise is *not* proof. Some of the so-called energy enhancers may give you a temporary surge like a cup of coffee or a candy bar would. But also like caffeine and sugar, your body will probably be *more* fatigued afterward. These "energy enhancers" may work in a pinch, but they are external solutions to internal imbalances. They mask your fatigue for a while, fooling you into thinking you have more energy. But the fatigue is still there, just waiting for the adrenaline rush to be over.

If women aren't going from health food store to health food store searching for energy enhancers, then they are going from doctor to doctor looking for a medical cause of their fatigue. Although it's true that fatigue is a symptom of almost every illness and that prolonged exhaustion can sometimes be an indicator of diabetes, cancer, heart disease, sleep apnea, low thyroid functioning, low blood sugar, iron deficiency, depression, mononucleosis, allergies, fibromyalgia, or chronic fatigue immunodeficiency syndrome, the vast majority of the time fatigue is simply fatigue—a warning sign from your body that something is amiss and out of balance. More energy is being expended than is being replenished—and you'd better refuel quickly. And as you will discover, a woman's fatigue warning system is more advanced and more persistent than a man's. Our brain chemicals, hormones, and blood supply are all involved in making sure that we "feel" our fatigue, acknowledge it, and do something about it.

When you *feel* tired, accept the fact that you *are* tired. Your body is communicating with you—trying to get your attention about the fuel gauge approaching empty and telling you that energy in is not equaling energy out. It's informing you that you have one of two choices:

1. Either *expend less* energy by doing less—taking a break, rescheduling an appointment, taking a nap, meditating for a while, saying no to unsatisfying obligations, canceling a date with a draining friend, or letting the laundry sit in the basket until tomorrow.

2. Or *replenish more* by eating a nutritious meal, having a snack, drinking a glass of water, taking a brisk walk, getting a good night's sleep, inhaling a few deep breaths, basking in some sunshine, or inviting some intimacy, fun, laughter, and play into your life.

Actually you do have a third (and most effective) choice: Do less *and* energize more. But I don't want to overwhelm you with too much before you even get into this book. We'll take it one small, non-fatiguing step at a time. Many women argue that they absolutely, positively, hands-down cannot under any circumstances do less. They have homes, businesses, churches, organizations, infants, toddlers, teenagers, partners, employees, employers, parents, in-laws, siblings, friends, and pets who are depending on them. Will the house clean itself? Who's going to do the grocery shopping? Pay the bills? Submit the report? Complete the project? Chair the committee? Give the kids a bath? Supervise homework? Cook dinner?

Invest their parents' retirement funds? Help that friend in need? Take the dog to the vet?

Whether we're indispensable or codependent is a matter of debate. And we'll discuss that later. But for now, if you feel you cannot shed some things from your hectic life, you can still understand, acknowledge, and address your fatigue. You can still replenish the massive amounts of energy you're expending each day—simply and naturally—by tapping into your 8 sources of natural energy.

1. **Food: Sink Your Teeth into Caloric Energy.** To give 100 percent, you have to get 100 percent—all the calories, carbos, protein, fat (yes, some fat is energizing!), vitamins and minerals, meals, and snacks you need to replenish your body.

2. **Water: Take a Sip of Hydraulic Energy.** Cool, refreshing, thirst-quenching water fights fatigue. When your body is water deprived, you're energy deprived. But when your body is properly hydrated, your energy is quickly restored.

3. **Fitness: Power Your Body with Physical Energy.** A strong, fit, muscular body has the power to run faster than a speeding bullet, leap across tall buildings, lift a powerful locomotive . . . well, maybe not quite . . . but it does have the stamina to react, think, problem-solve, carry the groceries, vacuum the house, and make it to your appointment on time—often with energy to spare.

4. **The Great Outdoors: Surround Yourself with Natural Energy.** Go ahead, fool with Mother Nature. Take advantage of her fresh air, sunshine, flowers, plants, rivers, lakes, mountains, and beaches. Then make your home and work environment pleasing to your soul and energizing to your spirit by bringing nature to you.

5. **Sleep: Recharge Your Battery with Restorative Energy.** Nothing restores the body and mind more than a good night's sleep, and a nap can be rejuvenating if it's short and satisfying.

6. **Intimacy: Tap into Your Sensual Energy.** Loving and being loved can fuel your soul. A close friendship, a loyal pet, a touch, a hug, a kiss, and, of course, passionate sex can all lift your spirits.

But being loving and kind to yourself may be the most powerful energizer of all.

7. **Joy: Tickle Your Soul with Comic Energy.** A one-minute laugh rejuvenates you more than a twenty-minute walk. A smile (even a forced one) can lift your mood. Being silly, playing jokes, and having fun is not just for kids—it's for your soul.

8. **Balanced Stress: Calm Your Chaotic Energy.** You can't live without stress, and sometimes it's a source of positive energy: anticipating a new challenge, getting excited about a new experience, or looking forward to a change in routine. But the negative stressors often zap our excitement: an overwhelming to-do list, endless obligations, and constant worry. Achieving balanced stress is the life-affirming goal.

When was the last time you focused on replenishing your energy with these 8 natural sources? When was the last time you enjoyed the taste of fat without guilt? Stopped everything and ate immediately when your body sent hunger signals? Sipped ice water on a leisurely afternoon? Walked on the beach to breathe in the fresh sea air? Drove to the mountains to behold the beauty of Mother Nature? Slept in an extra hour? Asked for a hug? Gave a hug? Made love in the afternoon? Laughed until you cried? Spontaneously called a friend for a drink? Done nothing without the guilt that you should be doing something?

If it's been longer than twenty-four hours, I strongly suggest that you stop everything right now and do one of the above to replenish your body. Instead of trying to override your fatigue by drinking coffee, taking supplements, ignoring it, working through it—outsmart it by recognizing what it is, what your body is trying to tell you, and what you need to do (or not do) to energize your body, mind, and soul.

Food, water, fitness, nature, sleep, intimacy, joy, and balanced stress—this is where real energy comes from; these are the areas in your life that will give you the vitality and enthusiasm you are searching for, not just for the next hour but for the next million hours. And you don't have to search any farther than your kitchen, bathroom, bedroom, family room, and backyard. They are within arm's reach, just waiting for your grasp.

OUTSMARTING
FEMALE FATIGUE

Chapter One

THE FEMALE ENERGY
CRISIS

When was the last time you were beside yourself with excitement and exploding with vitality? When was the last time you talked with a female friend or family member who boasted about her burst-at-the-seams happiness and endless supply of energy? When was the last time you encountered *any* woman who had an enduring bounce in her step, an enthusiastic smile on her face, and extra time on her hands?

Never? It's been so long you don't remember? For a fleeting moment last month? In a dream you had last week? For you, your friends, and 100 million other women, the positive feelings of excitement, energy, and happiness that used to regularly brighten our days seem to have vanished or at best are a rare, short-lived occurrence. And instead, the typical woman today is more likely to be beside herself with exhaustion, exploding with stress, bursting at the seams with frustration—and the only thing she's likely to have on her hands is calluses.

The indisputable medical fact is: Women are tired. Day after day in our exhausting struggle to do more and more in less and less time, 80 percent of us report fatigue. It's the most frequent complaint we bring to our doctors and the number-one topic of conversation with our friends. We're in an energy crisis—but most of us are too busy to do anything about it or too tired to even realize it.

Do you feel tired right now? Probably an unnecessary question. Whether it's 9 A.M. or 9 P.M., you may be struggling to keep your eyes open, trying to stifle a yawn, or having a difficult time concentrating on this paragraph. The fatigue that used to hit us once a day in midafternoon now hinders us morning, noon, and night. Perhaps the more appropriate question is: *How* tired do you feel right now? Mildly fatigued or full-body exhausted? On this scale of 1 to 10, evaluate your level of energy and rate your fatigue.

10 I'm exploding with endless, unstoppable, enthusiastic energy.

9 I could run a marathon, clean out my closet, pay the bills, and be done in time to pick up the kids from school.

8 I'm productive and efficient and can't wait to go to my aerobics class after work.

7 I'll push myself to make it through the day, but I'll crash tonight.

6 I don't think I can make it through the day; give me caffeine!

5 I'm falling farther and farther behind schedule—with no energy to catch up. Where did the time go?

4 I'm running out of gas, my battery's almost dead, and if someone asks me to do one more thing, I'm going to blow a gasket.

3 My eyes hurt, my feet are dragging, and my brain has gone off-line.

2 My life is completely out of control; I haven't had a break for months and probably won't get one until I'm six feet under.

1 I'm in a semiconscious stupor, unable to think, talk, or move.

Many of my clients let out an incredulous "HA!" at levels 9 and 10, questioning whether any women exist with "endless, unstoppable, enthusiastic energy." In contemporary society, this kind of daily stamina is a statistical improbability. But you may personally know one or two women who by all outward appearances seem to "have it all together" with their house, hair, career, and children always in perfect order—plus extra time left over to work out, take the newest kick-boxing and body-sculpting classes, volunteer in their kid's school, shop for the latest fashions, read the current best-sellers for their book club, fight for social changes they believe in, and keep their car sparkling clean.

But how similar is their life to yours and the average American woman? They may have a live-in nanny, a daily housekeeper, a professional chef to prepare meals, a personal shopper, a personal trainer, a personal assistant, and plenty of time on their hands as well as a professional manicure. Or they may not have the resources for this entourage of help, but they do have the facade of the "perfect, together woman" in public. In private, however, that facade may quickly fall apart as the hectic pace of life gets the best of them. Whether their outward energy is authentic or an illusion, these are the women we "love to hate"—the enviable exception to the rule. But I'd still bet a million dollars that behind closed doors they, too, feel overwhelmed and stressed, get hit with the three o'clock slump, and experience the fatigue that comes from the natural hormonal changes of PMS and perimenopause. As you'll discover, some fatigue is a normal and natural part of being a woman. But if by chance you are one of these "endless, unstoppable, enthusiastic" women (I didn't think so, but you never know) and rated your energy at levels 8 through 10, give this book to a fatigued friend. She'll thank you for helping her to outsmart her fatigue, and you'll be even more energized by your good deed.

If, instead, you chose levels 4 to 7, it might give you peace of mind to discover that you are a typical tired American woman and have plenty of company. According to the recent survey "The State of American Women Today," 67 percent of us report that we don't have the energy to make it through any given day. And even when we do manage to make it to the end of the day, we collapse into bed worn out, pooped out, burned out, and stressed out. This book was written for *you* and will help you realistically outsmart your fatigue so that you'll have the energy not only to make it through the day—*but to master the day with enjoyment, enthusiasm, and vitality.*

Now, if numbers 1 through 3 describe your state of fatigue, please do *not* put this book down. No matter how little time or energy you have, keep reading. This amount of fatigue is *not* typical, *not* normal—and *not* something you have to live with every day. What's most important is that you recognize the urgency of your energy crisis and begin to restructure your life by making a few simple changes to reenergize your body, mind, and soul—and revitalize your life.

Here's another telling question: How would you have rated your energy level five years ago? My research has found that 99 percent of women say they used to have more energy—before the baby, the stepchildren, the bigger house, the high-tech computer, the pager, the cell phone, the big promotion, the new at-home business, the ill parent, and/or the difficult divorce. And—before they stopped going to the gym, getting monthly massages, getting together with friends for dinner, going on vacations, sleeping in on the weekends, laughing at the lighter side of life, and generally taking care of themselves. Our progressive energy depletion is not just from the stress and work that's been added to our lives, it's also from the enjoyment and rest that's been taken away.

As I was researching this book, I surveyed over two hundred women on their level of energy, and their average level today is 4. Five years ago, they rated themselves at level 8. In half a decade, we've cut our energy in half and doubled our fatigue; we've gone from running to our aerobics classes to running out of gas. We've gone from feeling productive and efficient to falling flat on our backs. If we continue at the same unbalanced pace, what will happen five years from now? We won't be able to get back up. We'll be incapacitated by our fatigue with no energy left to break out of its binds. If we don't do something today to recharge our energy and outsmart our fatigue, we'll be walking around in a semiconscious stupor tomorrow not knowing what hit us.

FROM SUPERWOMAN TO STUPORWOMAN

One of my favorite clients, Susan, recently dragged herself through my office door with a self-diagnosis: "I know exactly what's wrong with me. I know why I'm stressed all day and can't sleep at night. I know why I'm so exhausted and unhappy. I have a chronic case of superwomanitis. Do you think my HMO will cover treatment?"

You may chuckle at this fabricated medical diagnosis because you know exactly what it means, but she was not making a joke of her life situation. She was dead tired and dead serious about it. "I do everything for everybody else and end up doing nothing for myself. I try to say the word 'no' but the word 'yes' slips out instead. I don't smile anymore. I don't have fun anymore. I don't have sex anymore. Twenty years ago, I bought into the superwoman mentality, thinking 'I can have it all, do it all, be all that I can be' . . . but the only thing I have is migraines, the only thing I do is play catch-up, and the only thing I can be these days is bone-tired. Well, I can't do it anymore! I'm checking into a secluded spa in the mountains tomorrow, and I'm never coming out."

Can I join you? Actually, a spa vacation isn't a bad idea. But if you're checking in to check out on life and get away from it all, the "it" will still be there when you get back—the frenetic schedule, the never-ending workload, the demanding boss, the screaming kids, the unappreciative partner, the unbalanced life, and the unrelenting stress. You can't run away from fatigue or escape from the responsibilities of day-to-day life, but you can validate your fatigue and acknowledge the busy realities of a woman's life.

- We work eighty-five hours a week between home and career—more than two full-time jobs!

- Over the past 20 years, we've added 158 hours to our annual job schedules and commuting times.

- We are responsible for over 90 percent of the day care, parent care, home care, healthcare, even pet care decisions.

- We do 1,473 hours of housework a year—the same amount we did in the 1960s when most of us didn't have an outside career.

- On average, we take only forty-five minutes to relax and unwind each night. And almost half of us say that our only true quiet time is in the shower or tub. The other half report that the car is their only sanctuary—when they're not taxiing their kids around town or returning calls on their cell phones.

With these statistics, it's no wonder that millions of us seek refuge in spas each year. We know that we can't continue at the same unbalanced, unhappy pace for much longer. We know we need a break, some R&R, a little pampering, a dose of healthy eating, some uninterrupted sleep, a fitness boost with nature walks, a mind/body makeover with meditation, yoga, and deep-muscle massage—anything to balance our stressed lives and rejuvenate us! But we also know that we need more than a few scheduled days of intense pampering in a spa—we need to welcome vitality back into our lives every day with the small, simple, and regular events that give us ongoing happiness and lasting energy.

For example, how long has it been since you:

had the uncontrollable giggles?

licked a lollipop?

dove in a pool?

went to bed an hour early?

played hooky?

soaked in a bubble bath?

took a nap?

wore a bright red "hey, look at me" outfit?

lingered at a candlelit dinner?

did a somersault?
ate chocolate-dipped strawberries?
watched the sun rise?

If you're anything like "Superwoman Susan" and my other clients, it's been way too long, maybe even since childhood for some of these simple pleasures or at least since your honeymoon or last romantic vacation. Over the last thirty years, women have accomplished great strides in education, politics, business, and sports—but we've been so busy running departments, running companies, running for office, and running marathons that we've forgotten the simple pleasures of walking on the beach, walking into the kitchen for a nourishing snack, or walking into the bedroom for a little nap or a little nookie. Then, on top of it all, while we've been focused on making history, making money, and making the world a better place for women, we're still making dinners, making babies, and making beds. We have no energy or time left over for making and keeping our bodies, minds, and souls healthy. And it's starting to take its toll on our well-being, health, and happiness.

- Only 24 percent of us can say that we live a "very good life"—down from 37 percent in the 1970s.

- Seventeen percent of women now experience migraines, up from 8 percent in 1970.

- The severity of PMS has increased fivefold in the last thirty years. Ten percent of us now experience PMS to such a debilitating degree that a new term, PMDD, premenstrual dysphoric disorder, is being used for diagnosis.

- Compared to the previous generation of women, our menopausal transition is five times longer, with double the hot flashes, double the memory loss, and double the weight gain. A new term has emerged for this heightened stage of female passage, too. It's called megamenopause—and 50 million baby boomers are struggling with it and wondering if it's ever going to end.

- One in four women will experience major depression in her life-time, up from one in seventeen in 1970. We may be *four times* richer than our grandmothers, but we're also *four times* more depressed.

Despair, pain, premenstrual dysphoric disorder, megamenopause, depression—are these the rewards for working so hard, doing so much, and being exhausted all the time? Some of us may have more money, a higher education, a bigger house, a nicer car, but the result-ing fatigue prevents us from enjoying our accomplishments and living life to its fullest. The National Institute of Aging recently found that regardless of success and good fortune over a ten-year period, we rated ourselves as no happier. So even if our schedules and bank accounts are filled to the brim, our lives are still lacking in fulfillment.

I hope that your fatigue has not reached this level of disharmony and unhappiness, but even if it has, look at it as a sign that your body is crying out for you to stop, reflect on your life choices, and redirect your attention to nurturing your body, enhancing your happiness, restoring your vitality, recharging your energy, and jump-starting your life.

IS YOUR BATTERY GOING DEAD?

Your body is really like a battery—it's a powerful energy source that can store energy, give energy, or "go dead" when its juice has run out. Luckily, it can also be jump-started and recharge itself. In order for your battery to last longer, burn brighter, and be continually recharged, the energy you give to your body has to at least equal the energy you're expending. In other words, energy in has to equal energy out.

ENERGY IN = ENERGY OUT

But for four out of five women, it doesn't. The vast majority of us are trying to expend massive amounts of energy with minimal amounts of fuel—and our batterylike bodies are running on fumes and about to go dead. If you're plagued by daily, relentless fatigue, there's an imbalance in your energy equation, too. The energy you're taking in doesn't come close to the energy you're putting out.

energy in < **ENERGY OUT**

I'm sure that you're quite familiar with the massive amounts of energy you expend day in and day out: the chores, the errands, the work, the growing in-box, and the expanding to-do list. But you may not be familiar with the energy you expend to simply be alive today: the energy it takes for your brain to handle 10,000,000 bits of information, or for your heart to beat 100,000 times, or for your lungs to breathe 25,000 times, or for your kidneys to empty 8 times, or for your digestive tract to move waste down its incredible 30 feet. You're expending even more energy than you think—both you and your body are working hard 24 hours a day.

Now let's look at the other side of the equation: the energy you take in to recharge your body, replenish your vitality, and provide the fuel for your body to live and function. Although food is the primary fuel for your body, the answer goes far beyond simple calories, vitamins, and minerals. Have you ever noticed how energized you feel after going for an invigorating walk on a bright, sunny day? Or after spending time with a good friend who has that contagious laugh? Or after a night of uninterrupted, restful sleep? Or after you've met an exciting new person or been to an exciting new place? Or after you've gotten a massage? Or after a great lovemaking session?

Food, exercise, sunshine, fresh air, sleep, laughter, new experiences, touch, and intimacy—these are the natural energy boosters that recharge your body, mind, and soul. These are what keep your energy equation balanced, your body functioning efficiently, and your life full of vitality. *These are the simple wonders that keep your batterylike body charged with positive life energy.*

In the most basic sense, energy is life. Each cell in your body is a living entity that requires fuel to produce energy. Your body is made up of an astounding 75 trillion cells! And each of these microscopic miracles is a tiny battery that needs nutrients, calories, water, and oxygen to produce the energy molecule ATP (which stands for adenosine triphosphate). The more ATP your cells produce, the more energy you'll have. To speed up ATP production, you can also make sure you get a good night's sleep, some exercise, some sunlight, some sexual pleasure, some laughter, and some positive stress. A fed, watered, oxygenated, well-rested, fit, glowing, sexually satisfied, smiling, and sufficiently challenged cell is a happy, healthy, and productive cell.

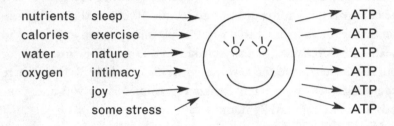

ENERGY IN = ENERGY OUT

Picture all 75 trillion cells in your body working efficiently for you by firing off ATP energy molecules. Imagine the energy you'd have in your body and the enthusiasm you'd have in your life. *The more energy you give your cells, the more vitality you give your life.*

How well are your 75 trillion cells? What does your energy equation look like? Is your battery juiced up and running efficiently, or is it about to go dead? Are your cells firing off ATP, or is your fire dying out? Think about today. Compare how much energy you've expended with the amount you've replenished.

Here's Lauren's reflection on her day: "The alarm went off at six o'clock, waking me from a night of tossing and turning. I dragged myself out of bed, felt my way to the kitchen to make coffee, jumped in the shower, and tried to get dressed before my kids got up. I made them breakfast and barely had time to blow-dry my hair before all hell broke loose when my youngest one decided to smear oatmeal all over the kitchen walls. Then I got them dressed, cleaned the walls, rushed into the car, dropped one child off at day care and the other at school. I looked at the clock, realized I was going to be late for my morning meeting, pushed the gas pedal, then got pulled over for a speeding ticket. I ran into the office a half hour late, had no time to go to the bathroom, and realized I hadn't eaten anything yet. During my meeting, my stomach was growling, my bladder was bursting, I couldn't think, and I kept squirming in my seat. By ten o'clock I was a basket case and there were over twenty messages in my in-basket. I had to run errands at lunch, so I didn't eat, which was fine with me because I'm trying to lose weight. When my three o'clock slump hit, I had a diet Coke and two Snickers bars. On the way home, I picked up the dry cleaning, stopped at the grocery store, bought a birthday card for my mother-in-law, picked up the kids, made dinner, fed the kids, ate dinner, bathed the kids, supervised homework, read bedtime stories, paid the bills, did the laundry, ate a pint of Chubby Hubby, then passed on my husband's advances to pass out on the couch at ten o'clock."

Sound familiar? What should be an atypical, hectic, crazy day is sadly a typical recurrence for many of us. What energy did Lauren take in? Caffeine, candy bars, one dinner meal, and ice cream. She didn't exercise, rest, sleep well, drink water, have fun, or have sex. But she did expend huge amounts of energy with her kids, job, errands, and other responsibilities and stressful activities. She was also trying to lose weight, which may be the biggest energy zapper of all. Not only are we trying to be superwomen, we're trying to be svelte, slender superwomen. We skip meals, skimp on calories, and sacrifice nutrition in the name of weight loss. I'll go into great detail on the draining effects of dieting in the next chapter, but if we never started dieting, we probably wouldn't be in such an energy crisis today.

The bottom line is: For the minimal amount of fuel we put into our bodies, we probably have the right amount of fatigue. For the huge amount we do each day, we probably have the right amount of exhaustion. Whether we're twenty years old or seventy years old, whether we work at home or commute to the office, whether we're full-time CEOs or full-time moms—we have too much on our plates (and often not enough food). And if we're full-time workers *and* full-time mothers, our plates are cracking from the load and shattering right before our bloodshot, tired eyes.

HARRIED . . . WITH CHILDREN

W A N T E D :

Multiskilled, caring individual to work 24 hours a day, 7 days a week. No pension, no lunch hour, no breaks, no sick days, no paid vacation. No salary. No sleep for the first year. No solitude for the next 18. Only volunteers need apply.

This is motherhood. And 67 percent of all mothers with young children are in the workforce, some part time, others full time, some commuting 100 miles a day, and others running businesses from their homes. It shouldn't be humanly possible to accomplish what working mothers do in a day, but somehow, some way they find an ember of energy and manage to get the kids ready for school, meet their company's sales quota, get that bonus, get that promotion, plan this year's vacation, make the family's doctor and dentist appointments, serve as retirement counselors for their parents, offer career counseling to their partners, play marriage counselor to their friends—I could go on and on with the monumental feats working mothers accomplish every day, but I'm exhausted by just typing out this partial list of responsibilities, obligations, commitments, and roles.

Juggling a variety of roles in our lives does not have to be detrimental, and can actually add an immense amount of stimulation to our minds and satisfaction to our lives. Over the last few decades, a number of studies have reported that the more roles a woman has as mother, daughter, worker, and partner, the healthier and happier she is compared to those with fewer roles. So we say, "Bring it on! I can have 2.5 kids, a beautifully decorated home, a glorious career, a thin, fit body—and be a loving partner, a perfect mother, a caring daughter, the soccer coach, the chairwoman of the fund-raising committee, and the president of the PTA all at the same time." But then we're so beat that exhaustion clouds our potential happiness.

Variety may be the spice of life, but too many spices can ruin the experience. Whoever said "Statistics are like a bikini; what they reveal is interesting but what they conceal is vital" deserves credit. Some research may show that multiple roles make some women happier, but where are these women? And how many roles are too many? For some women, a half dozen roles may be too many and for others, not enough. The key factor is how much we *enjoy* our multiple roles. It's not the number of roles we play, it's the enjoyment and fulfillment we get from playing those roles. And most working mothers say they're just "too damn busy and too damn tired" to enjoy them. While they're coaching their daughter's basketball team, they're thinking about the annual report that's due tomorrow. While they're taxiing their kids to school, they're talking on the cell phone with their accountant. While they're on the phone with their mother in the evening, they're cooking dinner, emptying the dishwasher, and feeding the baby at the same time. I suppose we could feel good about our multitasking talent—but it prevents us from enjoying the present moment and reaping the benefits from our life roles.

In reality, the lifestyle of many working moms seems far from happy or healthy. Duke University Medical Center found that working women with children release more stress hormones than working women without children. Did we really need a study to prove that? "Stress" is the most widely used word in a woman's vocabulary. Our stress hormone, adrenaline, is at a high level from the moment we wake up until the moment we go to bed. We have family stress in the morning as we get the kids ready for school; we have occupational stress as we're dealing with deadlines, presentations, projects, promotions, and demotions; and then we have family stress again as we're dealing with housework, homework, and paperwork. Men's stress hormones have a very different daily release. They secrete more adrenaline from 9 to 5, but they also have a quick drop in stress, adrenaline, and blood pressure when they leave work. Cornell Medical Center found that a man's blood pressure fell as soon as he walked through the front door of his house, but that we have little or no decrease in blood pressure when our day job is over. Because, in the words of the acclaimed book by Arlie Russell Hochschild, our "Second Shift" has just begun.

A Boston University study was one of the first to uncover the truth about a woman's twenty-four-hour workload. Working mothers put in nineteen hours more a week than working fathers: The dads put in a "meager" sixty-six hours a week between office and home compared to our monumental eighty-five hours. We do three hours of housework a day; they do only seventeen minutes. Which explains why they have the time to watch an hour more of TV and sleep a half hour longer each night. But we have little time to rest, relax, and recharge our bodies. What this comes down to is that we work an extra month every year. And, if my math is correct, an extra six and a half years in our lifetime! I think you'll agree, the term "working mother" is redundant.

Of course we're exhausted from our monumental workload. But what are we doing about it? One recent survey found that when we're feeling stressed out, overwhelmed, and ready to run away and hide in a cave, only one in ten of us will ask for help to lighten our load. The other nine try to keep a stiff upper lip and bear the stress of work, home, family, and career—until that lip starts quivering and the stress and fatigue become unbearable on our bodies, minds, and souls.

Why don't 90 percent of us ask for help? Perhaps because we're expected (and/or we expect ourselves) to do it all. If we don't meet our own and others' expectations, then we'll feel that we've failed. Maybe our mothers did it without any help; maybe we're in an unofficial competition with our sisters for the "Mother of the Year" award; maybe we don't have the resources to hire help. But we can still ask for help. Seeking out assistance from family, friends, and partners to balance our lives is a sign of strength, not weakness. If we don't ask, it's highly unlikely that someone (your partner?) will step forward on their own to offer help.

I have come across a few exceptional men who voluntarily share house care and child care, but when the bathroom needs to be cleaned, who grabs the brush to scrub the toilet? When the bed needs to be changed, who washes the linens? When an appliance breaks down, who schedules the repairs? When there's a party to go to, who RSVP's and buys the gift? When a child gets sick at school, who gets the call? When an infant wakes up in the middle of the night, who crawls out of bed? When there's a parent/teacher conference, who's more likely to go? You get the picture; perhaps you live it every day.

As we were discussing the inequity between a man's and a woman's workload, one of my more spirited clients shared with me her universal woman's motto:

If it has tires or testicles, you're going to have a problem with it.

And it rang true for me, so I thought it might hit home for you, too.

THE EXHAUSTING BATTLE OF THE SEXES

Men can sometimes add more work, more frustration, and more fatigue to our daily lives. But in all fairness to them, perhaps they aren't aware of what they're doing. The latest gender research has found that men don't know when *they're* tired, so they probably don't know when *we're* tired and need a break either. While our brains are hardwired for emotional connection and communication, theirs are hardly able to recognize or verbalize how they are feeling. A man's analytical left brain works independently from his emotional right brain. His left brain can be busy solving problems, doing reports, facilitating meetings, and running the numbers—and his right brain may be trying to tell him he's stressed and exhausted, but his left brain is not listening. He just keeps working and working without a lunch hour or an afternoon break until he devours dinner and passes out on the couch at night.

How often have you heard a man complain that he's "in a funk," "stressed out," or "pooped"? How often have you witnessed a man dozing at his desk or struggling to keep his eyes open in a meeting? How often have you seen a man sneak to the candy machine at work for an afternoon pick-me-up? Not very often. But these are daily occurrences for us because our right brain is always keeping tabs on what our left brain is doing. The corpus callosum, which connects the left and the right brain, is a whopping 23 percent larger in our brains, and constantly monitors our workload and stress and tells us when it's time to take a break, eat a meal, have a snack, drink a glass of water, or inhale a deep breath of fresh air. Many experts believe this gender difference may be one of the reasons why we have a lower rate of heart attacks and a longer life span than men do. We live seven years longer because we are always aware of our emotional and physical needs. Men have an earlier death because they are seldom aware of how to take care of their needs. And they'd have an even earlier death without us to nurture their health and remind them to eat nutritious foods, take their vitamins, have their teeth cleaned, have their eyes checked, and have their annual physical exam. Research has just discovered that single men die *three years younger* than married men. Marital status makes a big difference in how long men live, but makes little difference in how long we live. Does this mean that they need us more than we need them? Maybe. It could also mean that we almost always know what they need, but they seldom know what we need.

Many women expect their husbands to know when they need a break, a hug, a bouquet of flowers, some quiet time, or a helping hand—but a study at the University of Pennsylvania found that men were 25 percent less accurate in identifying people's emotional states based on their facial expressions. So a face of fatigue might not be recognized as a need for some rest or a look of sadness might not be followed through with a nurturing hug. Perhaps the conclusion of this research is that instead of expecting men to know what we need, we need to clearly express exactly what we need—and make sure they are listening to every word.

Because, alas, listening is not one of their fortes either. The University of Pennsylvania study also found that when men's brains weren't analyzing, strategizing, and negotiating, they were wandering. When their analytical left brain was not busy working and men were asked to clear their thoughts for thirty minutes, the oldest part of the brain, the reptilian brain, was firing off messages about physical contact: Fighting, football, and sex preoccupied the men's wandering minds. When the researchers instructed the women to clear their minds, a more evolved portion of our brain was processing messages about complex feelings and communication relating to issues of the day.

Michelle was sitting on the edge of her seat, analyzing this complex brain information and nodding in agreement. "This explains everything. While we have a twenty-first-century brain, theirs got stuck in the Neanderthal era. While we're talking about our feelings, they're fantasizing about fighting and fornication. While we're communicating, they're conquering." And when I shared with her our heightened ability in communication—we use six thousand words a day while they only use two thousand—she jumped up and verbalized her excitement. "What an advantage! At the end of the day, we not only get the last word in, we get the last four thousand words in." I couldn't agree more. It is quite an advantage.

While we're celebrating the female brain, let me share a few more fascinating gender differences: As men grown older, they lose twice as many brain cells as we do, their brains shrink more quickly than ours, and they become more forgetful than we do. So, if he forgets your dinner date, birth date, or wedding date, you can now understand why and be a bit more forgiving because of his less evolved, shrinking brain.

FEMALE FATIGUE: A WOMAN'S BLESSING

Most of my clients usually feel quite superior after learning about the differences between the male and the female brain—and can't wait to go home and inform their husbands. But before you make your significant other read the last section, finish reading this chapter. There's more to feel superior about. Our biological advancement extends beyond our brains to our uniquely female bodies. We have the vital, life-giving functions of pregnancy and breast-feeding—and therefore have a highly advanced survival mechanism that insists we rest for strength, eat for energy and nutrition, and sleep for repairing and restoring our bodies. A woman's body is a miracle of engineering, and explanations exist for everything we experience: Food cravings are a way to direct us to the nutrients we need, hunger is a way to ensure adequate calories and body fat for fertility, and fatigue is a way to ensure proper restoration for our bodies.

Take pregnancy as an example. No other time in a woman's life brings greater food cravings, hunger, and fatigue. Why? Because it's imperative that we eat more and rest more to provide energy for the growing fetus. Another evident example is the heightened fatigue felt during the transition to menopause. As the body is trying to find a new balance in hormones, our fatigue is trying to slow us down to have the energy to complete this important stage of female passage.

Actually, fatigue is involved in every stage of female passage: puberty, PMS, pregnancy, and menopause. Fluctuations in our female hormones, estrogen and progesterone, during these times make us more in tune with our bodies and our fatigue. If you happen to be premenstrual or perimenopausal when you try to ignore your fatigue, all I can say is: Go home, lock the doors, replenish your body, and don't come out for a while. Certain expletives have been used to describe our altered state at these times, and I'd just as soon not add any credence to those descriptions.

Like it or not, fatigue really does have gender—and female fatigue is powerful, persistent, and almost impossible to ignore for long. But the power of female fatigue even goes beyond the stages of female passage and our larger, more connected brain discussed in the last section. Just in case we don't acknowledge our fatigue and follow through with reenergizing activities, our female bodies have backup fatigue messengers that make sure we "feel" our fatigue and do something about it. Our bodies also communicate with us via low blood glucose, low brain serotonin, and the low points of our biological rhythms.

Blood Glucose

You may be feeling the fatiguing effects of low blood glucose right now. If you haven't eaten since you got up more than four hours ago, a wave of exhaustion may be hitting you like a tsunami, and all of a sudden you can't think, move, or form complete sentences. When your blood glucose level drops, so does your energy and mood. Every single cell in your body relies on blood glucose for energy, but your brain cells are 100 percent dependent on it. In fact, your brain's *only* energy source is glucose. Without a sufficient supply, your brain protests and won't let you function. When we hit this all-time low, sugar is often the only word we can murmur, and we head directly to the candy machine. These intense sugar cravings are actually a warning sign that your fatigue is so extreme that mainlining glucose may be the only way to get your brain back on-line long enough to get you home to crawl under the covers and take a nap.

Brain Serotonin

A woman's sensitivity to brain serotonin levels is a relatively new discovery. Serotonin is our "feel good" brain chemical that provides calmness, serenity, and productive energy. When it drops, our mood and energy quickly follow suit. Research has found that a woman's brain serotonin level can drop as much as 40 percent lower than a man's—when we're exhausted, stressed, premenstrual, menopausal, or when we're deprived of sunshine, sex, sleep, food, or joy. And when we're all of these rolled into one, it's time to head for the hills. We're completely discombobulated (as my husband calls it), and our brains start screaming through the language of serotonin to eat carbohydrates (complex or simple and preferably chocolate), take a nap, laugh, get some sunlight, or have some sex—all of which boost brain serotonin levels and alleviate our fatigue funk.

Biological Rhythms

Our energy levels, like our menstrual cycles and moods, are cyclical. We always have and always will experience the ebbs and flows of energy—every day, every month, and every year. Ninety percent of all women rate mid- to late morning as their high energy time and midafternoon as their low time. Ninety-eight percent of all premenopausal women report the most energy in the first two weeks of their menstrual cycle and the least in the last two. And 85 percent choose summer as their most spirited season and winter as their weariest. Think about your own energy cycles. When does your energy peak? When does it wane? Or has the energy crisis reached such heights that you can't tell the difference any longer?

For many, our highs have taken a nosedive and our lows are hitting rock bottom. Our 3 P.M. slump feels like we're being sucked into a black hole, our premenstrual fatigue is like a thick fog, and our winter blues feel like a blackout. And the positive, productive energy we used to feel mid- to late morning is on hiatus, our two good weeks a month have become more like two hours, and our spring awakening doesn't fully blossom.

Why? From this chapter, you now know—because we're not listening to our bodies and recognizing fatigue for what it is: a signal from our bodies that it's breaktime, naptime, mealtime, snacktime, funtime, downtime. But we don't take the time! If we did take a break every day at 3 P.M., rest during our periods, and sleep more during the winter months, we wouldn't be in such an energy crisis—with 100 million women functioning at 70 percent of their optimal capacity.

We used to take the time. Not us personally, but our grandparents and/or ancestors. Afternoon naps used to be built into the day (and still are in some less fatigued countries). Women used to spend three days in total seclusion and peace during their periods. Some historical accounts theorize that women were banished to caves or to "red tents" during blood flow because they were thought to be unclean, untouchable, and cursed. Other interpretations argue that we were not cursed, but instead celebrated the opportunity to be alone to rest, relax, and remove ourselves from the chores of day-to-day living. The latter explanation makes a lot more sense to me.

In today's world, I sometimes wish there were caves and tents, but for the contemporary woman, there is little solitude and too much stress. We try to fight our three o'clock slump, ignore our premenstrual needs, and treat January no differently than July. We're in an energy crisis because we're ignoring our bodies' instincts and trying to fight our biological rhythms.

When written in Chinese, the word "crisis" is made up of two different characters: one for danger and one for opportunity. The energy crisis is telling us that we're in danger and can't exist like this for much longer—and it's encouraging us to use this warning as an opportunity to take action with changes that will bring our bodies back into balance.

So let's heed that warning and use our energy crisis positively. Our hormones, brain chemicals, blood sugar levels, and biological rhythms are encouraging us to take advantage of the positive effects of eating, exercising, sleeping, nature, sunlight, intimacy, and laughter. And when we do, our bodies will reward us with heightened energy, happiness, and vitality.

We may "feel" our fatigue more than men, but we also feel more energized and get a greater lift when we take the time to replenish our female bodies.

- We are five times more likely than men to have a boost in energy and mood after eating.

- We feel twice as energized after exercising, even though we start off feeling more fatigued.

- We have better eyesight and hearing at every age, allowing us greater stimulation from the visual beauty and the sounds of nature.

- We have a greater serotonin release from food, sunlight, laughter, and sex.

- We have ten times more touch receptors on our skin, making massage, cuddling, and foreplay more pleasurable.

"Now these are female facts to really get excited about!" Michelle exclaimed. "Fight fatigue with foreplay. Eat your way out of exhaustion. Lift energy with laughter." I hope that you, too, are excited about a new biologically based approach to enhancing energy. Excitement itself is energizing. And fatigue is an opportunity to harness all of our female energy and bring vitality back into our lives today, tomorrow, and forever. So let's all get excited and grasp the opportunity to create a powerful, happy, balanced, and peaceful future.

Chapter Two

FREEING YOURSELF FROM FATIGUE AND FINDING YOUR VITALITY WITHIN

If you didn't realize how tired you really were before starting this book, you now know that you're exhausted—and rightly so! If you didn't realize how urgently you needed to balance your energy equation and break free from the trap of fatigue, you now know that your body is anxiously awaiting its energy awakening. But how do you begin the process of solving your personal energy crisis and finding your vitality within?

The truth is: You already know. Instinctively, your body has been trying to guide you down the path of enhanced energy, vitality, and happiness. You just haven't been paying attention. Maybe you've been too busy to listen to your body's messages or too tired to follow its directions. And now you feel lost in the complicated maze of life or stuck at a dead end. Well, if you're at a dead end, turn around. If you're lost, get your bearings and consult a map—your body's detailed map to finding your vitality within.

Think about times in your life when you've felt your best, when things seemed to click and you were riding on a wave of positive life energy. What was different? The big difference was that you were paying attention, consciously or unconsciously, to your body and responding to its needs. You were doing the things you love with the people you love. You were physically active and emotionally satisfied. You were well rested and well nourished. You felt good about yourself, walked with confidence, and smiled with enthusiasm. Maybe you felt this way for a full decade or maybe only a few days—but the feeling was undeniable and unforgettable.

You can have this feeling back—and you can recapture it forever. But first, you have to open the lines of communication with your body. You have more healthy wisdom in your body than all the medical libraries in the world, and it's screaming to be heard. Your fatigue is trying to tell you *what* to do to feel alive again. Once you identify the "what," I'll help you figure out the "*how*"—how to make life-enhancing, fatigue-fighting changes that will solve your personal energy crisis—simply, naturally, and permanently.

WHAT IS YOUR FATIGUE TRYING TO TELL YOU?

This is an important question that I will be asking you throughout this book, and that I want you to ask yourself right now. Say the words out loud or write them down on a piece of paper:

What is my fatigue trying to tell me?

and then see what comes up for an answer. At different times of the day, you'll have different answers, and at different times of your life, you'll have different answers. *But what is your fatigue trying to tell you right now, this very moment of your life?*

If this is the first time you've attempted to explore the internal, deeper meaning of your fatigue, a few pitfalls can arise. You may have an extreme answer like Gayle did: "My fatigue is telling me that I need a new job, a new boss, a new husband, a new therapist. Basically, it's telling me that I need a new life." When we've fallen into the depths of fatigue, sometimes our first thoughts are to go to the other extreme and completely revamp our lives. While you may eventually come to the conclusion that a major life change is called for, you don't necessarily have to quit your job, divorce your husband, or run away to free yourself from fatigue. There's no guarantee anyway that the new job will be any less stressful than the old one, or that a new husband will be any more helpful than the old one. Your fatigue is not telling you that you need a new life; *it's telling you that you need a new outlook on life*. One that gives you full permission to take care of your body and make choices that will enhance your health and well-being.

The second pitfall is to immediately blame yourself, as Holly did: "My fatigue is telling me that I'm weak, out of control, not organized enough, and not disciplined enough. It's telling me that I'm a failure in life." Let's set things straight right up front: *Fatigue is not your fault*. With the amount you have to accomplish every day, no woman would feel organized. In the continuous marathon of a woman's life, even the Bionic Woman wouldn't have the stamina to go 100 miles an hour day after day without hitting the wall. Let go of any blame you may be feeling. Your fatigue is not telling you that you have a character flaw, a discipline problem, or an organizational impairment.

The third pitfall is to assume that you need megadoses of vitamins or the latest energizing concoction that's hit the market. When Laura thought about what her fatigue was telling her, she was convinced that she "needed ginseng, ginkgo biloba, coenzyme Q_{10}, super blue-green algae, and B_{12} injections." These and other so-called energy boosters are what we're told we need by the companies that manufacture them. But this is not your body talking. Your body doesn't even know that these pills, potions, and injections exist. You may feel a lift from some of these products, but the energy is not permanent. Like caffeine, they are an external means of revving you up for a while, but once the effect wears off, the fatigue will come back in full force. You may choose to use them to push through the next hour or two of the day, but your body wouldn't choose them to recharge itself for life.

The fourth and final pitfall is immediately jumping to the conclusion that you have a disease or illness that's causing your fatigue. Karen was convinced that her fatigue was telling her that she had a life-threatening illness. She spent three years going from doctor to doctor looking for a medical cause for her fatigue, only to find that she wasn't ill, just tired. In fact, her medical anxiety and her many appointments had made her even more exhausted.

There are a number of cases, however, in which fatigue may be telling you that it's time to make a doctor's appointment. I would be remiss if I did not provide a brief discussion of the major medical causes of fatigue. It's a symptom of almost every illness and by itself cannot be used for a diagnosis, but in combination with other symptoms, it may be a warning sign of an undiagnosed and untreated medical condition. My goal is not to make you anxious about your state of health but to alert you to the fact that there is a small chance your fatigue is telling you that you may have:

- **Anemia**—either iron deficiency anemia or pernicious anemia from a B_{12} deficiency. These can be easily diagnosed with a blood test and easily treated with diet and supplements.

- **Hypothyroidism**—the thyroid gland secretes thyroxin, a hormone that boosts metabolism and energy. "Hypo" means underactive, and an underactive thyroid can bring about sluggishness and fatigue, as well as weight gain, hair loss, dry skin, and a sensitivity to cold. Because hypothyroidism is ten times more common in women than men (especially in women over the age of forty), many health professionals are recommending thyroid screening via a blood test as a standard protocol during an annual exam. If you do find that you have an underactive thyroid, the gland and your energy can be effectively boosted with medication.

- **Diabetes**—when insulin (the hormone that transports glucose from our bloodstream into our cells) is either low or ineffective, our cells are being deprived of energy. Other signs include excessive hunger, thirst, and urination. When diabetes is controlled by diet, pills, and/or insulin injections, our cells and our bodies are energized by a sufficient supply of glucose.

- **Hypoglycemia**—the opposite of diabetes, too much insulin can make our blood sugar drop below normal. Low blood sugar levels make us low in energy, but by keeping blood sugar levels stable through dietary changes, a more stable level of energy can be achieved.

- **Sleep Apnea**—what was once thought to affect only older, overweight men is now recognized as a potential problem for both genders at any age or weight. Often accompanied by snoring, sleep apnea occurs when we periodically stop breathing for as much as twenty seconds due to blocked airway passages. The lack of oxygen at night can cause lack of energy during the day. A number of techniques, devices, and medications are now available to help minimize this condition.

- **Adrenal Gland Insufficiency**—this is a relatively new term in the medical literature. After years of chronic stress, the adrenal gland can become worn out and produce low levels of the stimulating hormones, cortisol and epinephrine, causing lethargy. Effective treatment is still being researched, but balancing hormones and reducing stress appear to be at least part of the solution.

- **Clinical Depression**—fatigue is definitely one of the warning signs of depression. But it's one of those chicken-and-egg situations. Which came first? Did the overwhelming fatigue cause the depression or did the depression cause the fatigue? Sometimes it's impossible to know. But if you're depressed, don't waste time trying to figure it out, and instead take the time to take care of yourself through cognitive therapy and/or antidepressants. Every good therapist will help you make changes in your life situation to boost your happiness and your vitality.

- **Chronic Fatigue Immunodeficiency Syndrome (CFIDS)**— what used to be more simply called chronic fatigue syndrome has been expanded to recognize its immune involvement. It is accompanied by symptoms other than fatigue such as muscle pain, sore throat, tender lymph nodes, and memory loss. A diagnosis is difficult, and generally, if the fatigue decreases daily functioning by 50 percent, is not lessened by rest, and persists for at least six months, then along with the presence of the other symptoms, a diagnosis is made. This is not a book for CFIDS sufferers, but the recommendations given may still help.

• **Fibromyalgia**—characterized by painful muscles, tendons, and ligaments, fibromyalgia can also cause constant fatigue and recurring headaches. A diagnosis is often made by assessing pain when applying pressure to the eighteen "tender points" on the body. One of the best treatments to date is pain management.

Fatigue can also be a symptom of mononucleosis or the Epstein-Barr virus, cancer or heart disease, arthritis or allergies, Lyme disease or digestive diseases. Again, please don't let these potential medical conditions alarm you too much. The chances are slim that you have one of these health problems, but at the same time, however, I also don't want you to completely disregard the possibility. If you think that an underlying health problem may be the cause of your fatigue, I urge you to consult a skilled, empathetic physician and have some screening tests to identify a potential illness or rule it out. Even if you don't think an illness is your culprit, after reading this book and implementing the recommended changes, if you still find yourself at the same level of debilitating fatigue, make an appointment with your physician for a thorough exam.

So now you know that your fatigue is *definitely not* telling you that you need to get a new life, blame yourself, or take external and unnatural "energy boosters." And you know that your fatigue is *probably not* telling you that you need to identify and treat a major illness. Next, I want to help you figure out what your fatigue *is* really trying to tell you—the universal answers to your female energy crisis, the choices you make every day in how you live. Your fatigue may be begging you to make other choices to take care of your body from the inside out. Your body may be telling you that it desperately needs to be replenished by one or more of the 8 natural energy sources:

1. **Food: You need to sink your teeth into caloric energy.** A meal or a snack, some carbohydrate, some protein, or (are you ready for this?) some fat. Inadequate fat intake causes inadequate energy. Low calories cause low energy. Food is your body's primary energy source, and eating is a woman's foremost and immediate energy stabilizer.

2. **Water: You need to take a sip of hydraulic energy.** Dehydration is one of the top causes of fatigue for women, so heightened energy may be just a few glasses away. Cool, refreshing, thirst-quenching water hydrates all 75 trillion cells, especially your brain cells. Your brain is 75 percent water! So a water-deprived brain is an energy-deprived brain.

3. **Fitness: You need to power your body with physical energy.** An out-of-shape body can lead to out-of-this-world fatigue. Only 20 percent of us exercise consistently enough to power our muscles, hearts, lungs, and entire bodies. The rest of us would experience at least a 25 percent jump in energy if we jumped off the couch to move our bodies.

4. **The Great Outdoors: You need to surround yourself with natural energy.** Get some sunshine, breathe some fresh air, take in the beauty of Mother Nature. The sights, smells, and sun are immediately invigorating. Hiding from the sun and the outdoors with sunblock, sunglasses, and sun hat is hiding from an important energy source. We're all concerned about skin cancer and premature aging, but ten minutes with Mother Nature is all you need.

5. **Sleep: You need to recharge your battery with restorative energy.** On average, we're getting only 80 percent of the sleep we need each night, and when we're in menopause, it can drop as low as 50 percent. Sleep allows your body to repair damage, recover from stress, and restore balance. A good night's sleep leads to a good, productive day.

6. **Intimacy: You need to tap into your sensual energy.** Time spent with friends, lovers, children, and animals is rejuvenating time. But time spent being loving and kind to yourself may be the most energizing of all. The more confident and assured you feel about yourself and your body, the more pleasure you'll get out of every waking moment.

7. **Joy: You need to tickle your soul with comic energy.** Smile! Laugh! Snicker! Snort! Giggle! Guffaw! We need it; half of all women say that they feel sad at any given moment, so part of our fatigue may be our sadness talking, telling us we're emotionally drained from despair, worry, guilt, and anxiety. Laughter can help lighten our mood and lift our energy.

8. **Balanced Stress: You need to calm your chaotic energy.** Daily, chronic stress keeps us running around in circles with no reprieve. The only way to break free from this chaotic madness is to purposefully slow down, make it a priority to rest, and consciously choose where you expend your energy.

These are your 8 natural energy sources that are always at your fingertips. When you grasp them, they are your 8 energizing strategies to lifelong vitality. Sometimes your body will tell you it needs more of one strategy than another—but together these strategies are your solution to outsmarting your female fatigue!

It's very possible, however, that your body is telling you one overriding, very important energy secret and has been since you were a teenager. It's begging you to do something that will positively affect each of the 8 energy sources. For some women, this is all they need to do to free themselves from fatigue. What is that energy secret?

PLEASE, OH PLEASE, STOP DIETING

If your body could talk to you, it would plead with you to have more common sense and better judgment when it comes to dieting. It would probably sit you down for a heart-to-heart talk on the dangers of dieting, saying something like "Please don't do it! Don't ignore my hunger signals! Don't starve, take those pills, follow that ridiculous plan, watch that infomercial, or be tempted by that "guaranteed weight-loss" program. The refrigerator's full, the cupboards are stocked, and the grocery store is down the street, so please eat! You're an educated woman with enough smarts to know that the less you eat, the less energy you'll have and the more I'll slow you down to conserve fuel. I'll have no other choice than to steal calories from your muscles, decrease your metabolism, slow down your brain waves, stimulate fat storage, and do everything I can to survive."

But our bodies' pleading goes in one ear and out the other. We become the rebellious dieter, going against the centuries-old maternal wisdom of our bodies. We think that we know better than our bodies. That this next diet will be the miracle solution, and once we lose the weight, we'll be happy, energetic, and successful. Losing weight may very well be what your body needs if you are carrying more weight than is healthy for you. A bigger body can zap your energy. It takes more effort to move, lift, stand, and walk. It takes more energy to simply make it through the day. But as I'm sure you know from past experience, dieting is not the solution to weight loss. In fact, the opposite is true: Dieting is a major cause of our weight gain. Each time we've dieted, our weights have climbed—and the average American woman is now twenty-five pounds heavier because she's dieted. So we're tired not just from the energy lost by dieting, but also from the weight gain that's caused by dieting. Your body is trying to let you in on a little secret: "Guess what? If you stop dieting, I'll help you lose weight *and* gain energy at the same time."

Let's fast-forward ten or twenty years. As women mature, they gain a better respect for their bodies' wisdom. As you grow older, you will have wished that you took your body's secret to heart and stopped dieting today. "If I knew then what I know now . . ." is a common phrase used by our elders. Well, you do know now. Your body knows. You don't need to wait a decade or two for that wisdom to surface. You have the internal wisdom to stop dieting today.

For the 50 million women dieting right this very second, listen to what your body is desperately trying to tell you: *Stop Dieting!* You're only adding another layer of exhaustion because of the fat-storing, energy-depriving, dehydrating, weakening, asphyxiating, self-esteem-zapping, joy-robbing, stress-inducing effects of dieting. *Dieting is draining all 8 of your natural energy sources.* Here are the fatiguing facts of the dieting doldrums:

1. **Dieting cuts calories.** Sometimes fat calories are the enemy, other times it's carbohydrate calories, and often it's all calories. We skip meals, eliminate whole food groups, vow to never eat a morsel of fat again, and take diet pills to suppress appetite—then pray that weight loss will follow. We spend weeks in self-starvation eating low-fat, low-calorie foods. How much energy do you think your body can derive from cabbage soup, bran muffins, grapefruit, or iceberg lettuce? Not much.

2. **Dieting dehydrates the body.** When we try to lose weight quickly, much of the weight we lose is not fat weight, it's water weight. The high-protein diets especially cause you to lose body fluids because the uric acid end product needs to be excreted through your kidneys—and takes water along with it. And any low-calorie diet will cause you to make more frequent visits to the bathroom as your body tries to flush out ketones, acetones, and other waste products of self-starvation.

3. **Dieting decreases body strength.** Within forty-eight hours of dieting, you start to lose muscle mass, which is your metabolically active tissue. And less muscle means less strength, stamina, and energy. Even if we exercise while we diet, some muscle loss and energy loss is inevitable. And if we exercise too much because we look at it as another way to "burn" more calories, our muscles become overstimulated, and we become overtired.

4. **Dieting decreases oxygen consumption.** As our bodies work to conserve calories in every possible way, our breathing rate slows down and becomes shallower. We take in less oxygen and

therefore become less able to oxygenate our brains and cells. Less oxygen equals less energy.

5. **Dieting interferes with sleep.** A recent study in the *American Journal of Clinical Nutrition* found that dieters took 70 percent longer to fall asleep and enjoyed only 75 percent of the deep, restorative sleep of non-dieters. Diet today, and you'll have sleep problems tonight.

6. **Dieting decreases intimacy, sensuality, and self-esteem.** Dieting and body hatred go hand in hand. The more diets we've been on, the greater our body dissatisfaction and the lower our self-esteem. Dieting also prevents us from spending intimate time with lovers and quality time with friends. Who wants to go to a romantic restaurant when all you can order is salad with the dressing on the side? Who wants to go to a party when you can't eat or drink anything?

7. **Dieting decreases joy.** It's not much fun following a strict meal plan that's devoid of your favorite foods. It's even less fun when we go off the diet and gain the weight back, plus some. Once we get caught in the depressing cycle of on again/off again dieting, food guilt, weight worries, and weight preoccupation start to consume our thoughts—and we feel stuck in the psychological trap of dieting. In addition, dieting has recently been found to reduce brain serotonin levels, which causes even greater mood swings and more sadness. Any way you look at it, dieting is a downer.

8. **Dieting increases stress.** All of the above effects of dieting cause stress, plus dieting itself is a physiological stress. It causes an adrenaline release in response to the life-threatening situation of self-starvation. This is why some women say they feel "high energy" when they first start a diet. Your body wants to make sure that you have the energy to search for food for survival. But it's hyper-emergency energy, not calm, natural energy—and eventually you'll hit the diet doldrums with a fatigued body and brain.

After hearing these fatiguing facts about dieting, many women are in a quandary. "But I know I have too much weight on my body, and I need to lose it for my health. If I don't diet, what do I do?" You take a slow, realistic, non-dieting approach to weight loss. Although it's not within the scope of this book to outline this natural and successful approach, I have written other books dedicated specifically to weight control for women. If you are under the age of thirty-five, I encourage you to read *Outsmarting the Female Fat Cell*. If you are thirty-five or older, *Outsmarting the Midlife Fat Cell* is the solution for you. These books will give you all the education, support, and guidance you need to reach a comfortable, healthy weight—without dieting.

I often fantasize about a world without dieting. No thin ideal, no self-starvation, no food guilt, no body hatred, no isolation, no eating disorders. It's a great fantasy—and it can become a reality when we listen to our bodies and say, "No more diets!" We'd be smiling women with more strength, stamina, vitality, and body acceptance—and we'd have more time to develop ourselves and our lives. According to a survey by *Glamour* magazine, we spend one third of our lives preoccupied with our bodies—worrying about our weight, fearing weight gain, and struggling to decide what we will and will not eat. Without dieting, just think of the extra time we'd have to move, play, socialize, explore, sleep, rest, and develop our creativity and talents. Just think of the extra time we'd have to tap into our 8 natural energy sources.

THE 8 ENERGIZING STRATEGIES

Are you ready to dive deeper into what's really causing your fatigue? Are you ready to identify what you need to do to outsmart your female fatigue and find your vitality within? To recap, the 8 energizing strategies to lifelong vitality are:

1. Food: Sink Your Teeth into Caloric Energy
2. Water: Take a Sip of Hydraulic Energy
3. Fitness: Power Your Body with Physical Energy

4. The Great Outdoors: Surround Yourself with Natural Energy
5. Sleep: Recharge Your Battery with Restorative Energy
6. Intimacy: Tap into Your Sensual Energy
7. Joy: Tickle Your Soul with Comic Energy
8. Balanced Stress: Calm Your Chaotic Energy

Your next step is to assess which of these strategies will be most important for you with the following questionnaires. Complete them with honest "yes" or "no" answers and you'll begin to get a picture of where to prioritize your efforts.

STRATEGY 1: FOOD
DO YOU NEED TO SINK YOUR TEETH INTO CALORIC ENERGY?

	yes	no
1. Is losing weight more important than gaining energy?	___	___
2. Do you often skip meals?	___	___
3. Is "eating enjoyment" something you haven't experienced since the Reagan administration?	___	___
4. Was your only break today at McDonald's (or other fast food establishment)?	___	___
5. Do you eat salad for lunch three or more times a week?	___	___
6. Do you feel uncomfortably full after eating lunch or dinner?	___	___
7. Do you eat the same foods day in and day out?	___	___
8. Are your cupboards and refrigerator stocked with fat-free foods?	___	___
9. Are you restricting calories to lose weight?	___	___
10. Do you rely on sugar for an afternoon boost?	___	___
Total number of "yes" answers	___	

If you answered five or more of these questions "yes," then you have much energy to gain from eating. Food is the first strategy and the longest chapter because what we eat (and don't eat) and how we structure our eating has a profound influence on how we feel. Undereating makes us underproductive; overeating makes us over-tired; eliminating almost all fat eliminates an important energy source; and dieting drains our energy.

Most women have a complicated love/hate relationship with food. We love food and can derive much pleasure and energy from eating, but we also loathe the calories and fat and fear the potential weight gain. Have no fear! This strategy will help you gain energy from food *without* gaining weight.

STRATEGY 2: WATER
DO YOU NEED TO TAKE A SIP OF HYDRAULIC ENERGY?

		yes	no
1.	Is water something you keep only in your radiator?	___	___
2.	Do you drink more than two cups of coffee a day?	___	___
3.	Is your urine bright yellow and concentrated?	___	___
4.	Do you sweat easily?	___	___
5.	Do you have night sweats and/or hot flashes?	___	___
6.	Do you live in a hot climate?	___	___
7.	Are you likely to quench your thirst with soft drinks?	___	___
8.	Do you drink more than one alcoholic beverage a day?	___	___
9.	Do you drink less than three glasses of water a day?	___	___
10.	Do you drink water only when you're thirsty?	___	___
	Total number of "yes" answers	___	

If five or more answers are affirmative, then dehydration is one of your fatigue culprits. One study recently found that dehydration was the primary cause of fatigue for women—we're drinking less than two cups of water a day. What about all those water bottles we're carrying around? It could be that they're more of a statement about fashion than about our well-being. Carrying doesn't necessarily mean we're drinking!

Plus, if you're experiencing menopausal hot flashes and night sweats, those dampened clothes and soaked sheets can reflect a one- to three-cup water loss. Add to that the sweat lost when you work out and the water lost when you drink coffee and alcohol—and you'll realize that our bodies are water deprived. Think about what happens to your skin when you don't drink enough water. The outer layer of cells shrivel up and die. Your other cells may not meet an early death from dehydration, but they do lose their moisture and shrivel up, and are unable to perform the biochemical reactions that give you lasting energy.

STRATEGY 3: FITNESS
DO YOU NEED TO POWER YOUR BODY WITH PHYSICAL ENERGY?

	yes	no
1. When the 1980s fitness boom hit, did you hide in the nearest fallout shelter?	____	____
2. Do your legs feel like rubber after walking up a flight of stairs?	____	____
3. Would you rather diet than exercise?	____	____
4. Do you circle the parking lot in search of a close spot?	____	____
5. Would you rather have liposuction than start an exercise program?	____	____
6. Will you find any excuse not to exercise?	____	____
7. Do you belong to a gym but haven't begun to get your money's worth?	____	____
8. Do you make New Year's resolutions to start exercising but never follow through?	____	____

	yes	no
9. If a friend asked you to go for a walk, would you suggest going for a drink instead?	___	___
10. Does watching someone else exercising tire you out?	___	___
Total number of "yes" answers	___	

If you answered at least five of these with a "yes," then fitness will be a key strategy for boosting energy—a greater key for you than for him. Women feel twice as energized after exercising as men do. In fact, a ten-minute walk around the block energizes us more than a candy bar. It's true; even a short bout of exercise is better than sugar. What if you eat ten candy bars instead of exercising for ten minutes? Sometimes we'll try to find any excuse not to exercise. But there really is no valid excuse.

Starting and maintaining an exercise program is one of the most difficult feats for us to accomplish. The average woman stops exercising within three weeks of starting. My goal will be to make you well above average by starting slowly and choosing the best exercises to make your energy flow. If you think of your body as an engine, exercise is your tune-up. It lubes your joints, takes the knocks and pings out of your muscles, increases the horsepower in your heart, and gives your body better gas mileage.

If you happened to answer "no" to all of these fitness questions, then I have a few more for you:

- Do you exercise eight hours or more a week?
- Do you feel guilty when you miss an exercise session?
- Do you exercise even when you're not feeling well?
- Do you exercise at the expense of spending important time with family and friends?

If too little exercise isn't causing your fatigue, then too much may be. Your body can take only so much on the running trail, on the bike path, or in the gym. Overexercise is becoming a bigger concern as more and more women replace compulsive dieting with compulsive exercising. Too much of anything, including exercise, isn't healthy. Exercise can power your body, but overexercise can leave you powerless.

STRATEGY 4: THE GREAT OUTDOORS
DO YOU NEED TO SURROUND YOURSELF WITH NATURAL ENERGY?

	yes	no
1. Is your idea of experiencing nature watching the Discovery Channel?	____	____
2. Do you consider yourself more of an indoor type of person than an outdoor type?	____	____
3. Is your breath of fresh air from your air-conditioning?	____	____
4. Is black your favorite color?	____	____
5. Do you work in a cubicle?	____	____
6. Do you live in a large city?	____	____
7. If you were to look out your window, would you see concrete?	____	____
8. Do you stay at home on weekends playing catch-up?	____	____
9. Is your primary outdoor time between your house and your car?	____	____
10. Do you try to completely avoid the sun by covering up with sunscreen, sunglasses, and sun hat?	____	____
Total number of "yes" answers	____	

With five or more affirmatives, you need more of what nature has to offer: fresh air, sunshine, plants, scents, colors, and beauty.

And if you can't go to nature, then bring nature to you: gardens and plants at your home and office, pictures of landscapes, tapes of ocean sounds, or wind chimes at your window. One natural element you can get regardless of where you live (unless it's the Pacific Northwest in winter) is sunshine. Let the sunshine in and feel the fatigue go out. Ten minutes is all you need to lighten your mood.

STRATEGY 5: SLEEP
DO YOU NEED TO RECHARGE YOUR BATTERY
WITH RESTORATIVE ENERGY?

	yes	no
1. Does it take longer than ten minutes for you to fall asleep?	____	____
2. Do you dread going to bed?	____	____
3. Has it been more than ten years since you've replaced your mattress?	____	____
4. Do you wake up more than once a night?	____	____
5. Do you go to bed worried?	____	____
6. Do you wake up anxious?	____	____
7. Is your biggest meal of the day at night?	____	____
8. Do you travel across time zones more than once a month?	____	____
9. Are you a night person?	____	____
10. Do you drink coffee or other caffeinated beverages after 3:00 P.M.?	____	____
Total number of "yes" answers	____	

A score of five or more means that a lack of sleep is keeping your vitality at bay. More than half of all women report a sleep deficit, especially new mothers and menopausal women. Before the invention of electricity, we got ten hours of sleep a night. Today we get an average of seven. How much sleep did you get last night? Even if it was just one hour less than you needed, you're functioning at two thirds of your optimal alertness today.

If what you need is a good night's sleep, this important energizing strategy discussed in chapter 7 will help you determine how many hours you need to feel rested, will give you the tools to catch up on lost sleep, and will outline the most effective techniques to fall asleep and stay asleep.

STRATEGY 6: INTIMACY
DO YOU NEED TO TAP INTO YOUR SENSUAL ENERGY?

	yes	no
1. Would you use a word like "disgusting" to describe your body?	____	____
2. Are you more concerned with having buns of steel than a heart of gold?	____	____
3. Has it been more than a week since you've gotten together with a good friend?	____	____
4. Has it been more than a day since you've talked with one of your good friends on the phone?	____	____
5. Has it been more than a week since you've had sex?	____	____
6. When you meet a new dog, are you likely to avoid contact with it?	____	____
7. Do you stand or sit with your arms crossed?	____	____
8. Do you fear bathing-suit season?	____	____
9. Are you more likely to shake a hand than hug a body?	____	____
10. Do you wake up most mornings "feeling fat"?	____	____
Total number of "yes" answers	____	

If you marked at least five with a "yes," you are not alone. I've sadly discovered that most women score too high on the intimacy questionnaire. After forty years of the thin ideal and dieting, our body image and self-esteem are lower than ever. Ninety percent of us dislike our bodies, one-third of us report that our body dissatisfaction prevents us from having sex, and one quarter of us report that feeling uncomfortable with our bodies prevents us from socializing with close friends. Our sensual and sexual energy is trapped beneath body dissatisfaction. The strategy discussed in chapter 8 will focus on the energizing effects of feeling good about ourselves and our bodies—and being with people and pets who bring out our positive energy. Vitality attracts; spending time with gregarious, happy, vital people always makes us feel good.

STRATEGY 7: JOY
DO YOU NEED TO TICKLE YOUR SOUL WITH COMIC ENERGY?

		yes	no
1.	If you were to look in the mirror right now, would you be scowling?	___	___
2.	Has it been more than an hour since you've laughed?	___	___
3.	Do you avoid smiling because of potential wrinkles?	___	___
4.	Do you feel a blank as to what makes you happy?	___	___
5.	Do you think it's immature to giggle?	___	___
6.	Do you think reading the comics is a waste of time?	___	___
7.	Do you think playgrounds are just for kids?	___	___
8.	Would you describe your sense of humor as lost and never to be found?	___	___
9.	Are you likely to feel sad more often than you feel happy?	___	___
10.	Do worry and guilt occupy your thoughts?	___	___
	Total number of "yes" answers	___	

At this point you know the scoring—and may find that your fatigue is telling you that there's a deficit of joy and laughter in your life. Laughter is an internal workout, increasing heart rate, blood flow, and breathing. It's also a stress reducer, decreasing stress hormones for up to thirty-six hours. When you're fatigued, it can be difficult to see the lighter side of life—but it is possible with a little effort and a lot of fun.

STRATEGY 8: BALANCED STRESS
DO YOU NEED TO CALM YOUR CHAOTIC ENERGY?

	yes	no
1. Do you believe that a woman's work is never done?	___	___
2. Do you work more than ten hours a day both in and out of the home?	___	___
3. Do you keep saying "yes" when you'd rather say "no"?	___	___
4. Has it been more than a year since you've taken a vacation, even a weekend away?	___	___
5. Are there not enough hours in the day?	___	___
6. Are you busy going nowhere?	___	___
7. Would you choose getting things done over getting together with a friend?	___	___
8. Is your calendar booked weeks in advance?	___	___
9. Are you either going 100 miles an hour or conked out with a dead battery?	___	___
10. Are you feeling guilty taking the time to read this book?	___	___
Total number of "yes" answers	___	

Chronic stress and debilitating fatigue are almost interchangeable. When we feel stressed, our body is stressed, and the fight-or-flight response cries out for recovery through fatigue, urging us to rest and replenish our bodies. But when stress never stops, fatigue never goes away. This is the last strategy because it's often the most difficult to implement. It's easier to add something positive to our lives through eating, exercise, sleep, nature, intimacy, and joy than it is to shed the negatives like stress, work, chores, and obligations. It's also last because the other changes that you make with the previous seven strategies will automatically calm your chaotic energy, relax your body, and make it easier to choose where you expend your energy.

What have you discovered from these eight assessment questionnaires? *You've discovered your own personal solution to lifelong vitality—that enthusiastic feeling of being alive today and always.* List the strategies from the highest to the lowest score, and you'll know where to prioritize your efforts.

1. _____

2. _____

3. _____

4. _____

5. _____

6. _____

7. _____

8. _____

What is making you so tired is also your secret to vitality—when you turn it around and use it to your benefit. For example:

If your energy zapper is:	Then your vitality booster will be:
dieting	eating
dehydration	drinking water

If your energy zapper is:	Then your vitality booster will be:
immobility	exercising
indoor imprisonment	Mother Nature
sleep difficulties	sleep enhancement
isolation	intimacy
body dissatisfaction	body acceptance
sadness	joy and laughter
too much stress	balanced stress

Let me give you a couple of examples of how these eight questionnaires directed some of my clients' efforts and helped them to outsmart their fatigue:

• Maggie scored highest on the food questionnaire, which didn't surprise her. She was on what she called her "lifelong lettuce diet." No breakfast, a salad for lunch, and a bigger salad for dinner, both with nonfat dressing. Her body and therefore her energy was in a calorie deficit almost every day. Her goal was to start small: to add some protein to her salads at lunch and dinner. Sometimes it was a diced chicken breast, or bay shrimp, or a hard-boiled egg. Then, after overcoming her fat phobia, she switched back to full-fat salad dressing. After a few weeks, she really got daring and had meat lasagna with real cheese one night for dinner. Within two weeks, she felt her energy lift, and within a month she had more energy than she had had for years without any weight gain.

• After filling out these questionnaires, Karen discovered that dehydration was draining her energy. She claimed that she hated the taste of water, and drank coffee and iced tea throughout the day. Plus, she had recently entered the menopausal transition and was changing her T-shirt three times a night because of night sweats. When she started with just one glass of sparkling water with a slice of lemon, she realized that it was plain tap water she didn't like. Then she worked her way up to five "lemon lifts" a day and estimated that she had lifted her energy level fivefold.

- Terry found that she was already maximizing her benefits from eating and exercising, but she scored highest on the intimacy and nature strategies because she "never saw her friends and never saw the light of day." She was a stockbroker, woke up before sunrise, worked in a hectic, windowless office, then went straight to her health club after work to exercise indoors. She was so exhausted by the time she got home that she seldom had the energy to socialize. Terry made just one change in her routine: She started walking outside with a friend after work. She got her socialization and sunshine at the same time.

These are just a few examples of how one or two simple changes can make a significant difference in how you feel. If you scored high on each of the 8 strategies, you'll still need to prioritize and make one small change at a time.

GOING INWARD BOUND

At this point in the education process, after exploring the female fatigue epidemic and the 8 strategies that will awaken our cells as well as our lives, my clients usually have one of two reactions:

1. Excitement. "I want to be enthusiastically alive instead of dead tired! I can't wait to start energizing myself with the eight strategies and start really taking care of myself. All my life, I've taken care of everyone and everything else. Now it's my turn!"

or

2. Resistance. "This all sounds great, but I don't have the time to free myself from fatigue! How can I find vitality and happiness when I can barely find the time to brush my teeth? How can I find the time to exercise when I don't even have the time to go to the bathroom?"

Which reaction do you have?

Let's address the resistance first. To be honest with you, it does take some time and energy to gain time and energy. Reading this book is taking time you probably don't have, and you may be distracted thinking about the six loads of laundry sitting in the basket, the ten messages that need to be returned, the dozen bills that need to be paid, and the three school lunches that need to be made.

But consider this: Think about how much time you spend (and waste) being tired. When you're tired, everything takes longer to do. It takes longer to make decisions, make it to work, make lunches, do the laundry, and pay the bills. A European study found that it takes 50 percent longer to complete tasks when we're exhausted. So here's my proposition: If you take the time to finish reading this book, I promise to give you the most time-efficient, simplest, and most natural ways to add permanent energy to your day and vitality to your life. No matter how busy your schedule, you can find a few minutes here and there to do something different and use the 8 energizing strategies to free yourself from fatigue.

It's not what you can't do, it's what you *can* do:

- You may not be able to go to the health club to work out, but you *can* find the time to walk around the block.

- You may not be able to get together with a good friend for dinner, but you *can* find the time to talk to her on the phone.

- You may not be able to get an hour massage, but you *can* do thirty seconds of deep breathing.

- You may not be able to go to the market for fresh produce, but you *can* keep a glass of water at your desk.

- You may not be able to take a soothing bubble bath, but you *can* smile at yourself in the mirror while you're brushing your teeth.

- You may not be able to drive to the park and sit among nature, but you *can* buy a plant for your desk at work.

You can do all these small, simple, energizing activities and more! *Think small and your rewards will be great.*

Now, if you're feeling excited—instead of resistant—about the prospect of recharging your body and boosting your energy, I still want you to think small. Take it slowly and progressively, and make sure that your goals are realistic. What are your goals? What do you expect to get out of this book? Let's go back to the energy scale from chapter 1 on page 2 to assess your goals.

Where are you now and where do you want to be? Suzanne was at level 3, but desperately wanted to be at level 10. "I always wanted to be a perfect ten, so I might as well try to achieve it with energy." I hate to be the bearer of bad news, but it's not possible to sustain endless, unstoppable, enthusiastic energy. You'll always feel some fatigue; you're a woman with biological rhythms, hormonal cycles, and an advanced brain. You might feel a rare level 10 every now and then, but wouldn't you be happy fluctuating between levels 7 and 8 with an occasional 9 and 6? If your goals aren't realistic, you'll never feel successful. If you don't have a plan of action to achieve your goals, you won't outsmart your fatigue.

With this book, you have a plan of action. The next eight chapters are your step-by-step plan that will help you successfully achieve your realistic goals. I will give you hundreds of ways to outsmart your fatigue and unlock your vitality—you get to pick and choose what works best for you based on your lifestyle, your personality, and your present situation. I strongly recommend that you pause after each of the next eight strategy chapters and practice the tips and skills you think will be most helpful for *you*. Not just for today or for the new year—but for the rest of your life.

From this chapter, you know what your fatigue is trying to tell you, you know which of the 8 energizing strategies will be most important in unlocking your vitality, and you know how to set realistic goals. Now it's time to get started.

It doesn't matter how long you've been in the energy crisis, how stuck you are in the trap of fatigue, how many diets you've been on, or how inattentive you've been to your female body in the past. What matters is how you approach life from this point forth. In the inspiring words of Mother Teresa:

> *Yesterday is gone.*
> *Tomorrow has not yet come.*
> *We have only today.*
> *Let us begin.*

And you can begin right now with the question that began this chapter:

What is your fatigue trying to tell you right now, this very moment of your life?

Whatever it is, close this book, take a break—and go do it!

Chapter Three

FOOD: SINK YOUR TEETH INTO CALORIC ENERGY

Clara called me up on the phone one afternoon, looking for advice on how she should eat to beat her fatigue. As she began to describe her situation, I could hear the exhaustion in her voice and the urgency in her words. "I'm tired twenty-four hours a day, but from two to four o'clock in the afternoon, I'm a complete zombie. It's three-thirty in the afternoon right now, and I'm about to collapse. I know I'm eating right, but something feels terribly wrong. I'm a very healthy eater, practically a vegetarian. I eat lots of fruits and vegetables throughout the day. I don't eat red meat. I don't snack. I don't eat fatty foods. I don't eat sugar. I don't eat refined breads, cereals, or pasta. I don't eat processed foods. That's why I'm so confused. How can I feel so tired when I'm eating so healthfully?"

Because the contemporary definition of "healthy eating" has overlooked general health. Preventing disease decades down the road has been the primary health goal, not preventing fatigue today.

Food has been scrutinized to such a degree that the immediate health and energy benefits have been overlooked or put on the back burner. "Less is best" has become the guiding principle of healthy eating: less fat, less sugar, less salt, less carbohydrates, less protein, less additives, less preservatives—and less food overall.

But *less food equals less energy.* The five major causes of "food fatigue" for women today have more to do with eating too little than with eating too much.

1. **We're not eating enough calories.** Right this very moment, 50 percent of us are restricting our calorie intake to lose weight, and if we're not restricting calories, we're eating too many "empty" calories from snacks and fast foods. Empty calories are low in nutrients and lead to an empty energy tank.

2. **We're not eating enough protein.** Despite the slew of best-selling "eat protein" diet books, many women still think that protein is bad and should be avoided.

3. **We're not eating enough fat.** Because 60 percent of us believe that everything we put into our mouths must be low in fat, we're gobbling up the 2,500 new fat-free products introduced last year, and many of our low-fat intakes are approaching unhealthy levels.

4. **We're not eating enough carbohydrates.** Many of us falsely think that carbos are hazardous to our health and our waistlines, and we've blacklisted high-energy foods such as bread, pasta, rice, and potatoes from our diets.

5. **We're not getting enough enjoyment, pleasure, and satisfaction from anything that we eat.** It appears that over half of us feel remorse with every morsel we put into our mouths. Guilt, not pleasure, describes the bulk of our eating experiences.

And too many of us, like Clara, have all five causes of food fatigue each and every day—which leads to a chronic, debilitating case of eating exhaustion.

As you begin this important chapter, try to clear your mind of society's so-called healthy eating rules and the "good food/bad food" debate. The rules are different when it comes to outsmarting your fatigue, and there are no bad foods when the goal is eating for energy. Much of my advice will go against what you may have read in magazines, tried to follow in other books, or heard on TV or the radio—and some of my recommendations may shock you.

Clara couldn't believe her ears when I told her that she was tired because her "healthy" eating habits were tiring her out, and what she needed to do was to eat more often, more calories, more snacks, more fat, more sugar, more protein—and perhaps most important, to eat more joyfully. "Now wait a minute! I've spent the last decade painfully cutting these things out of my diet. Now you're telling me to eat them again—and eat them with a smile on my face. I'll gain weight! I'll lose control! I can't do it! I can't follow such a radical approach!"

Yes, you can, and, no, this isn't a radical approach. It's a realistic approach that goes back to the basics of healthy eating: moderation and variety. Eat moderate amounts of a wide variety of foods regardless of their calorie, fat, and sugar content—and don't feel guilty about it. This philosophy can be traced back thousands of years to Hippocrates, whose wisdom taught us that the key to health was moderation in all things. And almost seventy-five years ago, a provocative book was written, *Diet and Personality*, that identified the eating habits responsible for causing fatigue and mood swings: skipping meals, eating too little or too much, eating a large meal at night, eating too quickly, feeling irritated at mealtimes, and being overanxious about food. These are the very same eating habits that are zapping our energy today—and the habits that this chapter will help you break to make your energy soar.

Are you ready to sink your teeth into caloric energy? Are you ready to boldly go where no woman has gone before? My first goal is to give you permission to eat—anything and everything in moderation—to outsmart your female fatigue and achieve your full energy potential.

THE ENERGIZER TUMMY

Food is your primary energy source, and your stomach is your primary fuel tank, letting you know if your energy potential is at full throttle or approaching empty. *What's going on in your stomach can either power your body or exhaust you.*

When your stomach is empty, your body's overriding goal is to get you to eat—to fill your energy tank and fuel your body. Your brain may have been focused on finishing that report or paying the bills, but an empty stomach distracts your brain from the task at hand and calls all forces to activate appetite and make you eat.

- Your stomach starts growling, churning, panging, gurgling, and rumbling—informing you that its current state of emptiness is not acceptable.

- Your mouth starts salivating—making you yearn for a delicious, mouthwatering bite.

- Your brain starts releasing powerful appetite-stimulating chemicals, neuropeptide Y and galanin—increasing your desire for carbohydrates and fat, respectively.

- Your blood glucose starts to drop—causing your 75 trillion cells to cry out for fuel.

These initial biological appetite triggers should force you to stop everything and eat. But we often try to fight them and delay eating until after we finish the report, run the errands, or lose another five pounds. If you don't respond to these appetite signals and stop to refuel your body within thirty minutes, your body's appetite center takes it up a notch and your eating triggers intensify.

- Your blood glucose drops to emergency levels and you are devoid of mental and physical energy. Your brain is in pain from glucose deprivation, perhaps giving you a raging headache, and the rest of your cells are suffering, too, because they can't make enough ATP energy molecules no matter how hard they try.

- Your stomach starts producing extra acid and you may get heartburn and/or an upset stomach.

- Your brain reduces serotonin levels, making you irritable and making calorie-packed carbos even more appealing.

- Your muscles start to break down their glycogen stores to provide some backup glucose for your cells, but depleted muscle glycogen also depletes your energy.

Once you've entered this second stage of appetite triggers, you may be nauseated, have a headache, get heartburn, and feel irritable and grumpy. Not to mention that you are absolutely famished, about to faint from hunger, and can't wait to get your hands on anything edible. All because you didn't respond to your appetite signals and energize your tummy.

Instead, let's assume that you do listen to your initial appetite signals and refuel right away. You'll feel energized immediately. As soon as the first bite of food makes contact with your taste buds, messages are sent to your brain, and your brain breathes a sigh of relief, knowing that food is on the way. The food then travels down your esophagus into your stomach, where it silences the gurgling and soaks up your stomach acids. As the first few mouthfuls enter your stomach and touch its walls, stretch receptors send more pleasing messages to your brain. "Hooray! She's not just biting, she's swallowing. I'm filling, and *everything* is proceeding according to plan."

Now your brain is really excited. It turns off the drop in blood glucose, halts the brain chemical changes—and alerts all 75 trillion cells to the pending energy boost that's just moments away. "Get ready for some glucose, amino acids, fatty acids, and nutrients! Get ready for an explosion of caloric energy!" To receive these benefits, all you have to do is literally sink your teeth into caloric energy.

But wait! Something's gone awry. These bites of food—they keep coming and coming. The stomach keeps expanding and expanding, and the stretch receptors start sending frantic messages to your brain. "Houston, we've got a problem. She's still eating, and I'm overfilling and reaching maximum capacity. Our plan is backfiring. Why is she still eating? Make her stop!"

Your brain's initial excitement quickly turns to disappointment. "Damn it! She's doing it again. She's eating that whole industrial-size package of fat-free crackers. Now I'm forced to switch gears. Instead of restoring her energy, I have to concentrate my efforts on storing all this extra food in her fat cells." So your blood supply is directed away from your brain and your cells to your stomach for labored digestion that could take six or more hours. And your fat cells are activated to get ready for storage.

Fat cells usually lie dormant, requiring little energy or attention. Unless we overeat—then they are called upon for their specialized function: to store, expand, and grow. As the next few hours go by, your fat cells are happily hoarding all the extra food while you are unhappily bloated and unbuttoning the top of your pants. Instead of the anticipated lift from eating, you feel lethargic. You can't focus, the unfinished report is still sitting on your desk, and you're starting to fear weight gain. When you overeat, *nothing* is energized—except your fat cells.

A little food gives you a lot of energy; too much food and your energy crashes. When you fill your stomach without overfilling it, you'll stop gaining weight and start gaining energy. Both undereating and overeating will prevent you from experiencing the energizing effects of food.

"But how much is too little and how much is too much?" Kim and all my other clients want to know. I've always answered this with one word—a handful. Less than a handful and you're not filling your food tank enough; more than a handful and you're filling it too much. *A good-size handful is all you need to fill your stomach without overfilling it, to fuel your energy without fueling your fat cells, and to lift your energy without making you lethargic.*

Kim's first thought was that she wished she had bigger hands. That may be your wish, too, but the reality is that your stomach is about the size of your fist, so a good-size handful of food becomes a fistful after you chew it. Kim's second thought was that this handful rule couldn't possibly apply to fat-free crackers, lettuce, carrots, fruit, nonfat cookies—or any other low calorie, fat-free food. Yes it can. Fat is the storage form of all food. When you eat too much salad, vegetables, fruit, pasta, crackers, and fat-free cookies, they are all converted to fat, and this same sequence of energy-zapping, fat-storing events will take place. The only way to prevent it is to eat every food moderately.

But after years of eating mega-portions in restaurants, jumbo servings at family meals, and supersize packages of snack foods and fast foods, most of us have what I call "portion distortion." Do you have it? Do you think a serving size is the entire package? Or a moderate meal is whatever you see on your plate? If so, your eyes really are bigger than your stomach and you're overeating. Here are a couple of standard serving-size shockers to help you reduce your eyes to the size of your stomach:

- three heaping tablespoons of ice cream (and not the whole pint)
- ten potato chips (and not the ten-ounce bag)
- a small hamburger (and not the Big Mac or Whopper)
- one half of a bagel (and not both halves with a half inch of cream cheese in the middle)
- one cup of cooked pasta (and not the pound package)
- one half of a sandwich (and not the whole foot-long sub)

All of these fit the definition of a moderate serving because they can fit into the palm of your hand. Your hand is the measuring cup of your stomach—so use it.

Before you start eating, assess whether the food could fit into your hand. Or, I guess you could use your hand to serve your portions, as Veronica did. It was a bit messy, but it worked for her, and she rationalized this technique by explaining, "My mother always told me not to eat with my hands, but she never told me not to serve with my hands."

There is one scenario in which a handful of food is not your solution to moderate eating—when your body gives you no request for food to begin with. Eighty percent of us eat when we're not hungry and when our stomach doesn't need to be energized with food. Do you? Many of us eat when we're feeling tired, thinking that food will boost our energy. So we reach for the cookie jar, open the refrigerator, or find ourselves in front of the candy machine. But if we aren't hungry, food won't energize us. Are you eating right now as you're reading this book, but your stomach already has plenty of food in it from the last time you ate, an hour ago?

"Fatigue eating" is a form of emotional eating. And women are more likely than men to eat for emotional reasons rather than biological ones. Studies have found that the only emotion men eat in response to is loneliness. We eat when we're lonely, too. As well as when we're sad, anxious, stressed, frantic, bored, tired, and depressed. We use food to escape our feelings, distract us for a few minutes, and numb our emotions. But a dozen cookies won't alleviate depression, fight fatigue, or silence stress.

I'm sure you've heard of the fight-or-flight response to stress. When we're up against a stressful situation, our bodies prepare to fight for our survival or take flight from the potential danger. Well, for many there is a third option: **fight, flight, or . . . *bite***. And we proceed to bite away our stress with mouthful upon mouthful of food.

When you're feeling stressed and/or exhausted, your body doesn't need to eat if you're not also feeling hungry. It needs something else to replenish your vitality—one of the other 8 energizing strategies. Maybe your body needs to move, or sleep, or breathe fresh air, or laugh, or drink a glass of refreshing ice water. This key question will help you to identify what you really need:

What is your fatigue trying to tell you right now?

If it's not telling you with hunger signals to eat, then eating will not replenish your energy and give you a boost. It will only stimulate your fat cells for storage.

To truly energize your tummy, keep these three points in mind:

1. If you're not hungry, no food will energize you—but one of the other 7 strategies will.

2. If you're hungry, eat as soon as possible to prevent your brain and body from going into the overhungry mode.

3. When you eat, consume a handful of food to prevent your body from going into the storage mode.

"But if I eat only a handful of food when I'm hungry, I'll get hungry more often and have to eat all day long!" Precisely. That's the way it should work; that's the way we were designed to eat. Snacking boosts stamina. *Small, frequent meals give big, long-lasting benefits.* This way, you're constantly fueling your body with a moderate amount of food that is never too much and never too little.

Society's "three balanced meals" approach can cause an imbalance in your energy level. With the quintessential breakfast, lunch, and dinner, too much time elapses between meals and too much food is eaten at dinner. This approach is based more on convenience than biology. The 9 A.M. to 5 P.M. work schedule (or 5 A.M. to 9 P.M. for those of us who are workaholics) doesn't allow for frequent snack breaks or frequent meals. And it doesn't coincide with your body's sleep/wake schedule. We are biologically designed to gather food and eat only when we are awake and active, from sunup to sundown. But Ben Franklin and the industrial revolution changed all that. With the invention of electricity, we now search for food and eat into the wee hours of the night.

The typical American woman consumes almost 1,500 calories from 6 P.M. on, with our after-work snack, large dinner, and after-dinner noshing. But our bodies need only 500 calories after day-light dims (and about 1,500 calories during the day). We're eating exactly the opposite of how our bodies want to eat for maximum energy, weight control, and health. If you're in your twenties, you may be able to tolerate the lack of calories during the day and the abundance of calories at night without adding too much weight or fatigue. But the typical forty-five-year-old baby boomer can't. Tufts University recently found that most midlife women can't burn off more than 250 to 500 calories at any one given time. Take our typical 1,000-calorie dinner: At most, 500 of those calories are burned for life energy; the remaining 500 are stored in our fat cells. We're stuffed from our large meals, and so are our fat cells. As we grow older, we're also growing wider from large, infrequent meals.

How many meals do you eat a day? The average woman eats only two and a half meals a day, not even the three balanced meals we're supposed to eat. If we double our meals, we'll double our energy. One study showed that increasing the number of meals, from three to five a day, increased work performance by over 40 percent! No other change gives this much of a boost, not even an extra week's vacation a year. With three meals a day, your energy can dip like a roller-coaster. But with five meals a day, your energy drops are barely noticeable, and you'll successfully help keep fatigue at bay. Here are some graphs to help you visualize the energy-stabilizing benefits of five small meals a day.

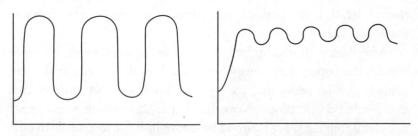

three meals a day   five meals a day

Because I don't want you to have an experience similar to Jackie's, let me be a bit more specific about the five *small* meals a day recommendation. Jackie didn't hear (or ignored) the word "small" and started eating salad, protein, starch, vegetable, bread, and dessert for every one of her five meals. After two weeks, she called me with an upsetting report: "This five-meal thing doesn't work for me. I feel worse instead of better. Not only am I more tired than I've ever been, but I've gained eleven pounds!"

The message is *not* to eat five courses in those five meals. It's to take the same food you eat in two or three meals a day and divide it up more evenly into five *small* meals a day. Have cereal for breakfast, fruit and yogurt midmorning, half your sandwich at lunch, the other half midafternoon, and a much smaller dinner. Use your hand to determine the definition of a small meal. And if all else fails, try hanging a mirror in your dining area. Researchers at Iowa State University found that when people saw their reflections in the mirror while eating, they ate a third less than those who weren't watching themselves eat.

If you still need more evidence for the benefits of five small meals a day, do your own research. Try it for a week and see what happens to your energy and your mood. Identify a friend whom you admire for her vitality and watch the way she eats. Or keep an eye on the eating habits of the real energy experts—kids. They would prefer to snack on small meals all day long—and have the energy to show for it. While you're at it, also observe animals. They graze throughout the day and always have the stamina to run, fetch, and play. Granted, they also take many periodic rest periods, but they venture over to the food bowl on a regular basis.

After Jackie cleared up her five-meal-a-day confusion, she experienced the anticipated energy boost and lost all the weight she had gained, plus an additional six pounds. Then she had another area that needed clarification. "Now that I know how much to eat in my five meals, tell me *what* I should be eating in those five meals to outsmart my female fatigue."

RATE YOUR PLATE

Your hunger will tell you *when* you need to eat to refuel and your hand will tell you *how much* you need to eat to reenergize. Now it's time to address *what* you need to eat to beat fatigue. Your body has the expertise to answer that question for you, too.

Sometimes your body just needs calories; it doesn't particularly care what kind of calories. Carbohydrate calories, protein calories, or fat calories will do the trick. Other times your body cares a great deal because it needs something specific to replenish your energy. It might tempt you toward fat for mood stability, or persuade you to go for a particular fruit or vegetable to get a nutrient for ATP production. Or it might vote for protein to build muscle, or push you toward carbohydrates to boost serotonin levels in your brain.

"But how do I know if my body needs carbos, protein, or fat?" asked Julie. "Some books and people say to eat more protein for power or to 'enter the zone,' whatever that is; others say to keep eating carbos for lasting energy; and now some are even saying to eat more fat. I feel like I'm stuck on a diet merry-go-round and don't know where it's safe to jump off. What do I eat? Who do I believe?"

Believe your body. No single type of food will be your fuel of choice all the time. Your body will need different foods depending on what's happening internally. And your body will let you know by making a particular food sound good to you, appeal to your taste buds, or satisfy your brain. In other words, you'll *crave* that food.

Up until recently, food cravings have been viewed negatively, as an uncontrollable weakness for an unhealthy food that must be fought with willpower. Not any longer. Food cravings are the *only* way for your body to communicate exactly what it needs to feel and function at its best. I helped pave the way to a healthier, more positive approach to food cravings with one of my books, *Why Women Need Chocolate*, teaching women that food cravings were normal, natural, and beneficial. And after almost a decade, many other health professionals are encouraging this approach and millions of women are embracing their cravings with a change in food philosophy: It's not the willpower to overcome your cravings; it's the "will" to "power" your body with the energy-boosting, mood-stabilizing foods your body needs.

Sometimes your body will need bread, or chicken, or steak, or spinach, or kiwi, or cantaloupe—and, yes, sometimes your body will crave chocolate because it needs chocolate. "Chocolate? If my body really needs chocolate, there must be a God." This was Julie's reaction to our discussion on food cravings, and she was elated to hear that chocolate increased "feel-good" brain serotonin levels. But whether you're experiencing a chocolate craving, an orange yearning, a pasta preference, or a meat urge, be assured that your body is sending you that message for a special reason, and you'll feel more balanced and energized after eating that food.

All you need to do is check in with your body to discover if it's craving any food in particular. Ask yourself the question: What is my fatigue trying to tell me to eat? What food or foods will be most energizing? Then follow through immediately by eating a small amount of it. Don't second-guess your body or question its expertise. It's telling you that you need a particular type of calorie (carbohydrate, protein, or fat) or a specific nutrient to recharge your battery.

The Eight Essential Energy Nutrients

Vitamins and minerals are not a direct energy source because they are calorie-free; only calories provide real energy for your body. But nutrients are involved in the biochemical reactions that make energy, store energy, sustain energy, or release energizing brain chemicals. All twenty essential nutrients are involved to some degree, but the following eight are the key players in encouraging your body to produce lasting energy.

1. **Iron.** This mineral is the most well known in fighting fatigue. A deficiency in iron, most common in women during the childbearing years, causes anemia. This decreases the amount of hemoglobin in

your red blood cells and prevents them from delivering oxygen to all your other cells. And without oxygen, your cells can't form ATP and you can't reach your energy potential. When your body and red blood cells need iron, you may crave red meat, legumes, dark green leafy vegetables, prunes, peaches, or watermelon. Surprisingly, watermelon is high in iron! And peaches can help iron out your fatigue!

2. *Vitamin B$_{12}$.* This vitamin is involved in red blood cell formation, and a deficiency causes another type of anemia, pernicious anemia. In addition, vitamin B$_{12}$ maintains healthy nerve function and aids in the production of "feel-good" brain chemicals. When you crave meat, fish, poultry, eggs, or whole grains, your body may be requesting B$_{12}$.

3. *Vitamin B$_6$.* With a long history of mood-stabilization properties, B$_6$ is involved in the formation of stress-calming serotonin and energy-producing ATP. When you reach for cereal, legumes, liver, and dark green vegetables, your body is thankful for the vitamin B$_6$.

4. *Magnesium.* This mineral is involved in over three hundred biochemical reactions in your body, including ATP and serotonin production. It is also a well-known muscle relaxant. A yearning for meat, spinach, or even chocolate may be due to a need for magnesium.

5. *Zinc.* This mineral boosts metabolism and calms anxiety, and it's the nutrient we're most deficient in—over 50 percent of us are not getting enough of it. Have you ever had a craving for raw oysters? It may be your body urging you to eat the food with the highest zinc content. Other foods with moderate zinc levels include meat, poultry, seafood, milk, and legumes. So when you have a yearning for these foods—think zinc!

6. *Chromium.* Another energy-boosting mineral, chromium helps to regulate and stabilize blood glucose levels by giving glucose molecules a push into your cells. If you've ever had a craving for a sandwich with meat, cheese, and whole-grain bread, it may be your body informing you that chromium is needed because this mineral is found in all three of these food groups.

7. *Boron.* This mineral helps maintain healthy mental function, including memory and attention span. If you forgot to eat your

boron and find yourself daydreaming, you may crave nuts, broccoli, or peaches or other fruits.

8. *Calcium.* Probably the most famous female mineral, calcium is not just beneficial for your bones, it's also needed to contract muscles and to calm the mind, especially during PMS. The *American Journal of Obstetrics and Gynecology* recently reported that calcium significantly decreased fatigue and fourteen other symptoms of PMS. Calcium is a leader in minimizing PMS *and* maximizing bone density. Along with weight-bearing exercise, calcium keeps your bones strong and resilient. Perhaps the phrase "bone-tired" should be taken literally. After years of not getting enough calcium, our bones become weak and porous. They tire more easily carrying the weight of our bodies around (as well as the weight of the world on our shoulders). So when your body craves milk, cheese, yogurt, or broccoli, say *"Bone appetit!"*

"But how much should I be getting each day of these eight energizing nutrients?" I could tell you that you need 1,200 milligrams of calcium, 1.6 milligrams of vitamin B_6, or 320 milligrams of magnesium—but I won't. Memorizing the numbers and adding up your daily intake would take too much brain space and take your energy away from simply eating a wide variety of foods, focusing on those that you crave.

"What about supplements? Should I take them?" I'll discuss supplements at the end of this chapter, and you may use them as a part of your food strategy to boost energy, but for now, think food first and think variety for vitality. By eating a wide variety of foods— breads, meats, legumes, dairy products, and vegetables and fruits— you'll fuel your body with the nutrients that it needs. The University of California at Berkeley reviewed data from the major national nutrition surveys and found that nearly one out of every two women aren't getting enough of just about every nutrient. So there's a fifty-fifty chance you're one of them and will feel revitalized by responding to your cravings, especially for fruits and vegetables.

Think produce for productivity. Fruits and vegetables are loaded with just about all of the energizing nutrients and are a surefire way to give your body a boost. Sneak veggies in whenever you can: Shred some carrots in your salad or tomato sauce, add some spinach to your lasagna or omelet, slice tomato for your sandwiches, or order pizza with vegetable toppings. You can also read *Stealth Health* by Evelyn Tribole for some other ingenious ways to add nutrition to your day.

But keep in mind that vitamins and minerals, in food or in pill form, do not provide direct energy to your body; they are indirect players in providing energy. Your real energy source is calories— calories from carbohydrates, protein, and fat. So, *instead of counting your calories, make your calories count.*

Pile Your Plate with Carbohydrates

Don't give in to the "carbos are hazardous to your health and your waistline" myth that's the rage right now. The pendulum is starting to swing back to center, where, hopefully, it will stay. Eating too much fruit, pasta, bread, cereal, crackers, bagels, pretzels, potatoes, rice, couscous, polenta, or corn isn't healthy for anyone. But neither is eating too much steak, chicken, pork, beans, eggs, or dairy products. During the 1980s and early '90s, we may have gone overboard with the carbohydrate pushing, but going to the other extreme with carbohydrate bashing isn't beneficial, either.

Starch, synonymous with complex carbohydrates, is broken down into blood glucose and provides fuel for all your brain and body cells. Without carbohydrates, you won't have the energy for your brain cells to think, your heart cells to beat, your lung cells to breathe, or your muscle cells to contract. You also won't have the ability to maximize brain serotonin release to stabilize your mood. When you eat starch, more tryptophan (an amino acid precursor to serotonin) is allowed through the blood/brain barrier and more serotonin is formed. And the benefit of starch on brain serotonin levels increases as we get older. Women over forty feel the calmest after eating a carbohydrate-rich meal.

At every age, carbohydrates make your brain and body happy and healthy. Trust your body and listen to your carbohydrate cravings, not to those pro-protein/anti-carbo evangelists who preach the evils of starch. While you're at it, also plug your ears when the pro-carbo/anti-protein group petition against red meat. Red meat in moderation isn't hazardous to your health, either, and can be as beneficial as a food of any other color.

Cultivate Your Carnivorous Side

Many of my clients are confused: Do they ask to pass the beef or should they pass on it? The answer depends on whether their bodies are craving red meat or other animal protein. When your body's not craving it, don't waste your time or your calories. But when your body is craving it, make haste and eat some protein right away. You'll feel immediately energized. Protein is broken down into amino acids, which in turn keep our muscles strong, our enzymes working, and our brains supplied with another important brain chemical, dopamine. Dopamine increases alertness and concentration—and keeps our brains working with maximum efficiency.

One of the primary causes of female fatigue is protein deficiency. Some of us may be eating too much protein, but many are still eating too little. Women who are concerned about fat, calories, and weight loss (the entire female community?) are more apt to choose the broccoli over the beef and the lettuce over the lamb. Or if we do eat animal protein, white is our color of choice: White fish, the white meat of chicken and turkey, and the other white meat, pork, are the only protein sources we allow in our diets. But sometimes our bodies need red meat and only red meat. No other color will do because our bodies are crying out for the combination of iron and protein to prevent anemia and outsmart our fatigue.

What if you're a devout vegetarian? There are other ways to supply your body with protein via dairy products, soy, legumes, and combining plant foods to get all the essential amino acids. But are you a vegetarian by choice or by force? Are you forcing your body to live a meatless existence when it would rather be eating meat? Some women are on "vegetarian diets," thinking that it is a healthier and more socially acceptable way to diet, cut calories, and fight fat.

Pass the Butter

Those three words, "Pass the butter," haven't been spoken boldly for a decade or more. If someone does announce from the end of the dinner table that they wish to place that yummy yellow spread on their bread, the other guests gasp in disbelief and give the speaker the evil eye. Then, as the butter is passed down the table to the daring diner, the other guests avert their eyes from the temptation and cast looks of jealousy at the butter eater.

This scenario may be a bit dramatic, but it makes the point that not only have butter and every other fat been shunned from the "healthy" dinner table, but we also negatively judge those who partake. I know because I've been the recipient of that judgment. I've always eaten some butter, salad dressing, deep-fried foods, and snack chips. Over the years, I've had clients run up to me at a hamburger joint as I'm placing a French fry in my mouth and yell "Gotcha!" I've had colleagues look into my grocery cart with shock at the potato chips, half-and-half, and butter, commenting, "I can't believe you eat that stuff." I've had friends prepare a supernutritious meal for the nutritionist who's coming to dinner, only to be speechless when they see the chocolate mousse truffle cake I've brought for dessert.

Okay, I fully admit it. I like fat. I crave fat. My body needs fat. If I don't give my body some fat every day, I'm dragging, out of sorts, and out of energy—until I have a handful of chips or another of my favorite sources of fat. You may crave fat, too. Most women do. Estrogen is made of fat, our brain cells contain fat, our nerves are lined with fat, our stomach requires fat to absorb the fat-soluble vitamins, our skin needs fat, and our happiness depends on fat. Fat has been found to release brain endorphins that elevate our mood and energy, producing a feeling of euphoria. Without it, we are depriving our bodies and brains of a vital energy source.

Both too much and too little fat are linked to fatigue, but from my experience with thousands of women, a low-fat diet is what's whittling away our energy. I would estimate that over 50 percent of my clients are depriving their bodies of fat. One of them is Jeannette. When she called me complaining of no energy, the first thing I found was that her diet contained virtually no fat. And the first thing I recommended was that she add some fat back into her diet. "You're telling me I should increase my fat intake? What kind of nutritionist are you?" I'm the kind of nutritionist who cares about the balance of your female body. I see a constant parade of women through my office, wanting to cut their already low-fat diet even lower. What they get instead is my help in increasing their fat intake.

My "eat some fat" recommendation has remained constant over the last twenty years. In the 1980s, as every woman's magazine, TV report, and health professional was warning you about the dangers of fat, I was warning my clients about the dangers of too little fat. I was also predicting that someday the tide would turn in fat's favor. And now it's starting to happen. There are research studies and magazine articles on the benefits of fat, and when women start reading about those benefits in *Cosmopolitan, Vogue, Self,* and *Redbook,* they finally start to believe it. And they start allowing some fat back into their diets.

STOP THE OIL EMBARGO

Fat is a nutrient. Like vitamin C, iron, and protein, it's something your body can't live without. But it's a nutrient society loves to hate, so we try to force our bodies to function on a low-fat diet, only to find that we can't function very well at all.

- A study from England found that when women cut their fat intake in half, their dispositions took a nosedive, too. They got angrier, moodier, and more hostile. Has your family been complaining about your hostile behavior? It could be due to your low-fat eating behavior.

- When you don't give your body enough fat, your metabolism slows down, just like when you're on a diet. Your body views it as a form of starvation, and you may actually start to gain weight as your body prepares for survival.

- A very low-fat diet has been found to cause failure to thrive—not just in infants but also in adult women. Some women are unable to maintain healthy body functions such as their menstrual cycles because of a deficiency in fat.

- The Harvard Nurses' Health Study, the largest research study ever on women, has followed eighty thousand women for over fourteen years. A recent finding is that those with the highest intake of monounsaturated fat (the "good fat" from olives, peanuts, and avocado) had the lowest heart disease risk. This study supports the heart-healthy benefits of the Mediterranean diet. Those living in Greece, Italy, France, and Spain have a high total fat intake but a low risk of heart disease because much of their fat comes from monounsaturated sources.

- What about the fat/breast cancer link? The Harvard Nurses' Health Study also found that a high-fat diet was not linked to breast cancer. The jury isn't completely in yet, but it appears you'd be better off focusing on eating more fruits and vegetables than on avoiding fat. Especially monounsaturated fat. A Swedish study recently found that those women with the most monounsaturated fat in their diets had one half the risk of breast cancer of those with the lowest intake.

- Plastic surgeons are even starting to see the negative effects of a fat-free diet: deeper lines, bigger bags, and looser skin. Some women are having fat injected under the skin to smooth out wrinkles that could have been prevented by including some fat in their lunch or dinner.

Mood swings, weight gain, failure to thrive, a higher risk of disease, and premature aging—these are just a few of the reasons why it's not healthy to live a fat-free existence. ***Following a very low-fat diet doesn't help you live longer. It only seems longer.***

When it comes to fat, we need the truth, the whole truth, and nothing but the truth. So what are the real facts about fat? First, we *all* need some. Second, most of us need more of the good fat, the monounsaturated fat. Monounsaturated fat is found in olives, olive oil, canola oil, soybeans, soybean oil, tofu, nuts, peanut oils, and avocado. So take that fat-free chip off your shoulder—and put some olive oil–based dressing on your salad, snack on some almonds, slice some avocado for your sandwich, nibble on some peanut butter and crackers, sauté some shrimp in olive oil and garlic, or dip some chips in guacamole. Your body will be thankful, and you'll be healthier, happier, and higher in energy.

Because the bathroom scale is often more important than our health, you may still be fearful of adding some fat because of potential weight gain. Have no fear! Fat in your diet does not become fat on your body—unless you eat too much of it. The best way to prevent eating too much fat is to stop dieting and restricting fat. The University of Toronto did an eye-opening, fat-revealing study. The researchers divided women into two groups: those trying to lose weight by restricting their fat intake and those not trying to lose weight. They gave each group a milk shake, then presented three pints of ice cream for a taste test. The group that wasn't weight-preoccupied had a taste or two of each flavor and walked away. The group focused on weight loss didn't budge until they ate through all the pints. This fat-restricting overeating response is called the "what the hell" effect. The weight-preoccupied women fell off the weight-loss wagon with the high-fat milk shakes, so what the hell, they might as well eat the ice cream, too, since they'd blown it anyway. Then, of course, their next thought is "I'll just starve myself tomorrow."

The best way to stop overeating fat is to stop restricting fat. When you try to eat fat-free, you'll make up for it with a fat binge later, eating high-fat foods all day long. This isn't good for your energy, mood, or health, either. You'll feel bloated and sluggish, and will almost be able to feel the fat clogging your arteries and brain. Some people call this a "fat hangover"—and it's a great image. Your body is trying to get rid of the fat, but can't deal with the truckloads of lard, oil, and butter you've just eaten. So it lingers in your system for hours.

If you use a bottle of olive oil to sauté your vegetables or eat a pound of peanuts this afternoon or go through a stick of butter a day— then yes, you'll gain weight and lose energy. But if you eat a moderate amount of fat, you'll gain energy *without* gaining weight.

What is a moderate amount? That's a difficult question to answer because it depends on your daily caloric intake, metabolism, and activity level. A ballpark estimate is to have somewhere around 30 percent of your total calories come from fat. If you're physically active, you can have even more. As an early plug for exercise, the more active you are, the more fat you can eat without compromising your health. Female athletes can have upward of 40 percent of their calories from fat, and the regular three-times-a-week exercisers can have 30 to 35 percent. But how do you translate that percentage into daily choices?

Generally speaking, one quarter of your food choices can be high in fat. Craving French fries today at lunch? No problem. Just balance the rest of your meal with three other low-fat foods, maybe a chicken breast sandwich with mustard, some carrot sticks, and a Popsicle for dessert. Want fettucine Alfredo for dinner? Go ahead, just make the next three meals low in fat. Think 3/4—for three quarters of your plate to be taken up with lower-fat foods, or for three quarters of your day to be made up of lower-fat food choices, or for three quarters of your week to be balanced out with less fat. Every single morsel that passes your lips doesn't have to be 30 percent fat calories or less, but that's the way we've interpreted the recommendation (or been told to interpret it). Instead, think about the average amount of fat in a meal, a day, and a week.

Are you ready to end the oil embargo that's been placed upon us by society? Start with a simple experiment and see how you feel. Take the next two days. Tomorrow eat the typical low-calorie, no-fat breakfast: 1 cup of cereal, 1/2 cup of skim milk, 1 cup of orange juice, and 1 banana. That's 360 calories and 0 grams of fat. On the next day, eat 1/2 cup of cereal topped with two tablespoons of almonds, 1/2 cup of 1 percent milk, and 1 cup of orange juice. That's the same number of calories, 360, but with 9 grams of fat, mostly monounsaturated from the almonds. Note the difference in your energy level, mood, and productivity. I'll bet you notice a significant difference— every woman I know has started gaining energy when she stopped her personal oil embargo.

While we're stopping the oil embargo, we might as well stop the sugar sanction, too. We've been eating sugar since the dawn of civilization. We can even trace our desire for sugar all the way back to biblical times, when Eve ate the forbidden fruit. Fruit is basically sugar. If you take away the fiber and nutrients, what's left is pure sugar, and your body can't tell the difference between that apple and apple juice, applesauce, apple pie, Apple Jacks, or an apple fritter.

It's impossible to achieve a sugar-free diet (fruits, many vegetables, and milk products all contain sugar), and why would you want to try? Some sugar can be a healthy part of your diet—it doesn't cause diabetes, trigger hypersensitivity, or go directly to our hips. Calories from sugar are not more fattening than calories from starch or protein. Duke University followed two groups of women who consumed the same number of calories, but one group ate a lot of sugar and the other ate very little. *Both* groups lost the same amount of weight.

I'm not necessarily advocating a diet high in sugar. Most of us consume too much to begin with, and we're eating more year after year. A new report from the Center for Science in the Public Interest shared some shocking sugar statistics. Since the 1970s, our sugar intake has increased by twenty-five pounds per person per year. Much of that increase is due to our soft-drink consumption. We drink fifty-four gallons per person per year—a 100 percent increase since the 1970s!

When you're craving sugar, your body obviously doesn't need pounds or gallons. A spoonful of sugar will help the fatigue come down. And a spoonful has only sixteen calories! Sugar causes a quick rise in your blood glucose level and a jolt to your brain, but unfortunately the energizing effects don't last very long, twenty minutes or a half hour at best. And then we hit an all-time low. With the sugar surge, your brain is initially happy, but the pleasure quickly turns to panic when your blood glucose level keeps rising. Sugar is a simple carbohydrate, which means that it's quickly digested and absorbed. Your brain wants to get that load of sugar into your cells, so it quickly releases large amounts of the hormone insulin from your pancreas. Insulin helps to transport glucose molecules from your bloodstream and into your cells, but when large amounts are released, too much glucose is carried into your cells. Then your blood sugar level plummets and your energy follows suit.

There is, however, a single foolproof, fatigue-fighting way to prevent the sugar high/sugar low: Don't eat sugar by itself on an empty stomach. Give it some company. Make sure there's something else present in your stomach that will slow digestion and absorption. For example:

- Have a glass of milk with that chocolate chip cookie—the protein will stabilize your blood sugar.

- Have a couple of crackers with those jelly beans—the complex carbohydrates will slow down the digestion of the sugar.

- Have a slice of cheese with that apple—the fat and protein will delay the absorption of the sugar.

- Have a little yogurt with those raspberries—the protein and fat will prevent the sugar low.

By giving sugar some company with additional starch, protein, and/or fat, you'll have lasting energy and a perked-up brain. There is no need to eliminate sugar from your diet. If you did, your taste buds wouldn't be very happy about it. Both sugar and fat have that "melt in your mouth" flavor that tantalizes your taste buds. And food flavor is an important, but neglected, energy source that you probably haven't heard of before. Your taste buds, however, can tell you all about it.

DO YOURSELF A FLAVOR

If you were blindfolded and taste-tested a rice cake, how would your taste buds react? And if your next bite was a luscious piece of European chocolate, how would they respond?

The chocolate would no doubt excite your taste buds, tongue, and mouth, sending thousands of pleasure signals to your brain. The sugar, fat, and five hundred other flavors would energize your senses and keep your mouth smiling. The rice cake, on the other hand, would be likely to make your taste buds yawn in boredom and put your tongue to sleep. If your husband, son, brother, or father did the same taste test, they would probably be bored with both the rice cake and the chocolate—and opt to grab a beer and turn on a football game for their stimulation.

We've already discussed a number of gender differences in this book—and taste is yet another where we come out on top. We have a stronger taste perception than men and are twice as likely to choose foods based on their sumptuous flavor. Because we get more oral and nasal satisfaction from food, some researchers call us "supertasters." This is why we love the foods that taste good to us and dislike the foods that leave a bad taste in our mouths. So, until someone invents broccoli that tastes like Ben & Jerry's or rice cakes that taste like chocolate cheesecake, we have to take our taste buds into consideration.

Don't get me wrong. I'm not suggesting that you forgo broccoli for ice cream or replace rice cakes with chocolate cake. But I am encouraging you to give pleasure to your taste buds. Happily stimulated taste buds lead to a happily excited brain. And we can acquire tastes for foods and beverages we once found displeasing. Many of us have done it with alcohol. That first sip of scotch made us cringe, but the more we drank it, the better it started to taste. We've also done it with artificial sweeteners. Their bitter aftertaste should have deterred us after the first diet soft drink, but weight issues prevailed and we trained our taste buds to tolerate the taste. If we can do it with Tab, Fresca, diet Coke, single malt scotch, whiskey, gin, vodka, beer, and wine—then we can do it with broccoli, cabbage, cauliflower, Brussels sprouts, wheat germ, and tofu, too.

But let's get back to chocolate and other flavors that are immediately satisfying. Just smelling and tasting your favorite foods can release those positive brain chemicals, serotonin and the endorphins. Actually, your nose may even be more instrumental than your mouth. Your olfactory senses can detect hundreds of variations in smell, and aroma is the first step in food satisfaction.

What flavors do your nose and taste buds favor?

- Chocolate? That simply means you're a woman. Chocolate is our number-one favorite food regardless of age, race, or body weight. With a blend of over five hundred aromas and flavors, no other food can compare.

- Hot foods over cold foods? Heat ignites flavors. Cooked foods are usually more pleasing to the taste buds than cold ones, and the Chinese have always adhered to the custom of eating foods that are cooked and then eaten warm. Not only do they taste better, but the Chinese also believe that cooked foods are more easily digested and maintain our energy flow.

- Spicy foods? Some women love hot and spicy Mexican, Hunan, and Indian food. Others like to add white pepper, black pepper, chili pepper, curry, onion, and garlic to their foods to make their taste buds tingle.

- Sour foods? Pickles, lemons, green apples, and sauerkraut can cause your taste buds to come alive.

- Salty foods? Our salt taste buds love to be stimulated; without salt, food can taste bland. Have you tried some of the flavorless no-salt breads or soups?

- Sweet foods? The term "sweet tooth" comes from the sixteenth century, and some of us have inherited more sweet taste buds than we'd like.

Our taste buds go beyond the four you may have learned about in biology class: salty, sour, sweet, and bitter. There is a fifth taste bud that may be the most powerful. The Japanese call it "umani," which means the *delicious taste bud*. We are calling it savory, a combination of flavors that's intangible and almost impossible to describe—but that is immensely satisfying.

To get the most out of flavors and stimulate your umani:

1. **Know your favorite flavors.** What are the flavors or combination of flavors that make all five of your taste buds happy?

2. **Don't waste your taste.** If you know you're looking for something salty, don't try to eat something sweet. It will never be satisfying to your taste buds or stimulating to your body.

3. **Let your nose join in on the fun.** Take a big whiff of the food before you start eating, then as you're chewing, close your mouth and breathe out through your nose. Chewing releases hundreds more aromatic chemicals.

4. **Don't bite off more than you can chew**—literally. Smaller bites stimulate your taste buds more than larger bites, allowing the food to spread evenly over the tongue.

5. **Slow down.** Chew thoroughly, savor the flavor, and let the food linger in your mouth.

6. **Focus on the first three bites.** These are the most satisfying to your taste buds and your brain.

If you follow the above recommendations, then theoretically, you need only eat three bites of any food to feel satisfied and energized.

By the time you take your fourth, fifth, or fiftieth bite you've maxed out the energizing effects from flavor, and your taste buds couldn't care less what you're eating.

Nancy decided to follow these steps with three bites of tiramisu. "My taste buds, body, and brain felt great for about one nanosecond, but then the guilt set in and I was in a funk for the next three hours."

TILT THE GUILT, TREASURE THE PLEASURE

Food fear, eating angst, gastronomical guilt, plate paranoia—most women know these feelings all too well. According to an American Dietetic Association survey, 50 percent of us feel guilty after eating anything. And when guilt sets in, the paralyzing worry prevents us from being energized by food. You may commit to eating more flavorful food combinations. You may focus on fulfilling your cravings for protein, fat, and carbohydrates. You may choose more nutrient-packed foods for the 8 energizing nutrients. But the most important thing missing from your plate may be pure, unadulterated enjoyment.

When was the last time you ate a meal free of guilt and full of pleasure? Your birthday? Last Thanksgiving? Your big job promotion two years ago? Your high school graduation twenty years ago? We can usually release guilt and fully enjoy our favorite meals on these and other special occasions, but when they are few and far between, we often eat too much because we know they are rare indulgences. I call this overeating response the "last supper syndrome": This may be the last bacon cheeseburger we'll see for a while, so we better eat two now while we have the chance. Then we might as well finish the entire cheesecake, too, because we may never have the opportunity to eat that sumptuous, fat-laden dessert again.

If we viewed every day as a special occasion and treasured the pleasure of every waking moment and every life-sustaining meal, then we wouldn't feel the need to overeat and would have no reason to feel guilty. But why don't we? The biggest reason is that we fear a bigger body. How can we enjoy a high-fat meal when we're trying to lose weight? Another major reason is that we're not encouraged to make eating enjoyable and food fun.

We can blame our government's dietary guidelines for the lack of attention to food pleasure; you won't find any mention of eating enjoyment in the USDA's recommendations. All other countries around the world recommend eating advice similar to ours: Eat plenty of fruits and vegetables and not too much fat, sugar, salt, and alcohol. But the one guideline other countries have that we don't is to eat with enjoyment and leisure and in the company of loved ones.

- In Great Britain, the primary message is to enjoy your food.
- In Japan, the connection between happy eating and a happy family life is emphasized.
- In Norway, health is viewed as a joyous combination of good food and good taste.
- In Thailand, a happy family is defined as one whose members eat together and enjoy treasured family tastes and good home cooking.
- In Vietnam, an emphasis is placed on providing healthy meals that are delicious, served leisurely and with affection, and eaten with family and loved ones.

When was the last time you and your family ate a delicious, leisurely, home-cooked, happy meal?

Happy meal? In this country, our only version of a happy meal is a colorful box picked up at a fast food drive-thru and eaten in the car on the way home. Leisurely meal? Breakfast always seems rushed, and our average lunch "hour" is twenty-nine minutes, barely enough time to go to the cafeteria or a deli. Dinner may be our most relaxing meal—when everyone is home from work and school on time, and when we're not rushing to make it to our evening meeting. Then we eat on the run and often in the car. So many of us now "dashboard dine" at the steering wheel that car manufacturers are responding with something that I would never have dreamed of. Within a decade, it has been predicted that some new cars will come equipped with microwaves. Will home cooking become a thing of the past? Will we start eating microwaved fast foods for breakfast, lunch, and dinner? I certainly hope not, but I do hope that we start enhancing our food pleasure and eating enjoyment—wherever we're dining.

You can follow every recommendation in this chapter to structure your eating for energy, but how you feel during and after your eating experience can either enhance your vitality even more or eliminate it. As with everything else you do in your life, if you don't enjoy what you're eating, you won't feel recharged from it.

VITALITY BITES

We've covered an almost overwhelming amount of information thus far, so let's simplify it and put it all together. Our best food choices are determined by a combination of our individual biological make-ups, our food cravings, and our taste buds. Other books may tell you specifically what to eat for the bionic breakfast, the rocket-launch lunch, the kick-butt dinner, and the warp-speed snack. But I won't because I can't. It's impossible for me to know your "vitality bites." I can only know mine, and mine are most likely very different from yours. I will, however, help you to identify your personal power foods.

To satisfy your curiosity, here are some of my top vitality bites: peanuts, potato chips, bananas, saltine crackers, bread, chocolate milk, yogurt, pizza, and mashed potatoes with gravy. As a comparison, I'll also share with you my sister's. A similar genetic structure, very different power foods: beef barley soup, potato leek soup, tomato soup, turkey vegetable soup, split pea soup, mushroom soup, chicken noodle soup, and French fries with gravy. At least we have one similarity: a potato product covered with fat. But other than that, I sometimes wonder if we're really related. I've witnessed her eating soup for breakfast, lunch, dinner, and a midnight snack—all on the same day. To tease her, I often call her the "Soup Nazi" (the character from that famous *Seinfeld* episode) because she's quite demanding and serious when it comes to her soup.

Actually, we should all take our power foods seriously. We must acknowledge them, covet them, and cherish them. What are yours? You can probably come up with a good list right now. After finishing this chapter, complete or revise this list to acknowledge at least twelve of your power foods.

1. _____

2. _____

3. _____

4. _____

5. _____

6. _____

7. _____

8. _____

9. _____

10. _____

11. _____

12. _____

Your vitality bites are usually quick and easy, always satisfying, and always rejuvenating. But think variety for lifelong vitality. The more variety in your vitality bites, the more energy you'll have and the more nutritionally balanced your diet will be. You need at least a dozen foods a day to ensure a varied diet, but if you're like most women, you eat the same limited foods day in and day out.

Do you eat the same thing for breakfast every morning? The same cereal, the same type of bagel, or the same cottage cheese on toast? Do you always go to the same deli for lunch and order the same salad or the same turkey sandwich with mustard only? Do you always order the chicken entrée in restaurants? Are the same foods on your grocery list week after week?

If you regularly eat fewer than a dozen different foods a day, then you need to branch out and add variety to your vitality bites. Experiment with different breads, gourmet pastas, dairy products, different cuts of meat, fish from around the world, and exotic fruits and vegetables. Eighty-six percent of us don't eat a single dark green leafy vegetable in a four-day period. When was the last time you ate kale, Swiss chard, spinach, bok choy, kohlrabi, escarole, radicchio, turnip tops, dandelion greens, mustard greens, cabbage, or Brussels sprouts?

The next time you go food shopping, add some new foods to your grocery list. Think seasonal and be creative to uncover some different foods that will unlock your vitality. Try sushi for lunch, Ethiopian food for dinner, or munch on a mango for a snack. Or how about having a sandwich for breakfast? It may be just what your body needs to fight fatigue.

What to Eat for Breakfast to Make Your Energy Last

Some women are hungry within minutes of waking; others aren't hungry for a few hours. First and foremost, let hunger determine your breakfast time. If you're one of those "I'm not hungry in the morning" people, you may also be one of those nighttime eaters who devour a triple-decker sandwich right before bed. If you eat late at night, you may falsely think your body doesn't need breakfast. Little digestion occurs while you sleep, so you'll wake up with a full stomach. Take a week and don't eat within three hours of bed; then you'll know your body's biological breakfast time.

Most women need a combination of carbohydrates and protein at their morning meal. Carbohydrates will replenish the muscle and liver glycogen that was used for energy while you slept (sleeping does burn calories) and will raise your blood sugar for the coming day. Protein will wake up your brain and release dopamine for a productive morning. So try putting some peanut butter or a poached egg on your toast or add some extra milk to your cereal for some extra protein. Or—have a ham and Swiss on rye and experience an energy high.

What to Eat for Lunch When You're in a Crunch

According to the National Restaurant Association, 40 percent of us don't even break for lunch. More and more of us are skipping lunch when there's more and more evidence that lunch is the most important meal of the day for women. Our metabolism is highest at midday, and that's when our bodies' need for refueling is the greatest. What are we doing at lunch if we're not eating? Forty-four percent of us run errands, 38 percent of us work, 27 percent of us shop, and 14 percent of us exercise (well, okay, you're forgiven for that one as long as you promise to eat something right after). So while we're not eating, we're running around expending more energy, which only makes us more tired in the afternoon. All nutritional studies have shown that when we skip lunch, we have greater fatigue, more migraines, and bigger mood swings for the rest of the day.

What's usually lurking in your lunch?

1. Nothing? If your lunch box is empty, your energy tank will be, too, and your three o'clock slump will be a permanent collapse.

2. A piece of fruit that you found at the bottom of your briefcase? Fruit is sugar, and by itself will cause the sugar high/sugar low— and make you less productive and sleepier in the afternoon.

3. A salad with nonfat dressing? Without protein or fat, your productivity won't last long. Within an hour, your energy will go sour.

4. A sandwich or a dinner-type entrée? Your body and brain will be in tiptop shape for all your afternoon activities.

A lunch that has some carbohydrates, protein, and fat produces the best results for afternoon stamina. Check in to see what your body is craving and focus more on that particular food, but also do a mental checklist of your plate to make sure your lunch has some carbos, protein, and fat. Even if you're only craving pasta, order a plate that has some chicken or shrimp in the sauce. Or if you're craving turkey, put a little mayonnaise or avocado or cheese on your sandwich for a dose of fat. A little fat gives you a lot of staying power by satiating your hunger for hours.

What to Eat at Dinner to Make Your Meal a Winner

Use two words to describe your typical dinner: Pepperoni pizza? Lean Cuisine? Big Mac? Takeout? Salad and salad? Cherry Garcia?

My client Annette chose Cherry Garcia, explaining "I'm so tired when I get home that I don't have the energy to make a nutritious meal. So I eat a pint of ice cream and pass out on the couch." When it comes to dinner, most of us are either too tired to prepare a meal or we're so famished from not eating during the day that we eat a huge evening meal followed by an ice cream dessert.

From this chapter, you now know that your body's caloric needs are minimal at night, so think of your dinner meal as your evening snack. If you've fueled your body throughout the day with small, frequent meals, it only needs a small handful of food at dinner anyway. But a handful of what?

Unless you work nights or have a deadline to meet by midnight, what you eat at dinner is probably the least important for outsmarting female fatigue. Your body should be tired at night because it's preparing for sleep. To help your body wind down for the night, eat light and focus on carbohydrates: pasta with tomato sauce, stir-fried vegetables over rice, or even a bowl of cereal. To wind your body back up and stay awake, eat mostly protein. A chicken breast, pork chop, filet mignon, small piece of fish, or scrambled eggs will provide dopamine for your brain and energy for your thinking. My only word of warning at dinner is to watch the fat—too much may hinder dopamine release or prevent sound sleep later that night.

What to Eat for a Snack When Fatigue Attacks

You can and should snack throughout the day. First, give yourself permission to snack. Second, make sure you're hungry. And third, check in with your body's cravings and identify what it needs for the best power snack.

Most of my clients virtuously inform me, "I only snack on fruit." Even though women snack on fruit more than any other food, your body doesn't always need fruit. And when it does say "Fruit, please" for your stamina snack, it won't always need an apple, our number-one fruit choice. In fact, if Eve had been looking for the healthiest snack pickings in the Garden of Eden, she would have chosen a kiwi over an apple. Apples don't give much to your body besides sugar and fiber, but kiwis, papayas, blueberries, cantaloupes, tangerines, mangos, and strawberries are packed with fatigue-fighting nutrients as well as disease-fighting phytochemicals. When you are craving fruit, be specific as to what kind and what flavor you're looking for— and make sure you give it some company with some protein or fat to stabilize your blood glucose levels.

Go nuts! Add some pistachios to your strawberry snack. How can nuts, something that's 70 percent fat, be good for you? Nuts are high in monounsaturated fat, protein, folic acid, and magnesium. The Harvard Nurses' Health Study found that five or more ounces of nuts a week reduced heart disease risk by 35 percent! So go ahead, nibble on some nuts.

Maybe with some chocolate? Chocolate with nuts is a great combination. Yes, chocolate can be a stamina-boosting snack choice— when you're craving it. Besides containing sugar, fat, and magnesium, it also contains phenylethylamine, which boosts your metabolism, alleviates depression, and mimics the feeling of falling in love. No wonder chocolate makes us feel so good. Let's chalk one up for chocolate!

While we're at it, we might as well give yogurt a snack award, too. Not only does it provide calcium, but it also contains a nice balance of protein and carbohydrates. But not all yogurts are created equal. With flavors like Strawberry Cheesecake and Mocha Latte, some contain more sugar than calcium or protein. And not all have lactobacillus, the active bacteria that has been found to aid in digestion and vaginal yeast infections. If that's why you're choosing yogurt, look for "live, active cultures" on the label.

And use your favorite yogurt to make a smoothie—the hip and popular snack choice. Most are made with low-fat yogurt, fruit, and skim milk, but others are made with ice cream and whole milk. The *University of California at Berkeley Wellness Newsletter* analyzed smoothies and found that they could have as many as 950 calories and 29 grams of fat! So keep an eye on what's going into the blender.

The possibilities for snack choices are endless. Anything from a slice of roast beef or pumpkin pie to a handful of potato chips or baby carrots. When you identify your power snacks, keep an emergency supply available at all times—in your purse, glove compartment, desk drawer, briefcase, gym bag, or jacket pocket.

Could an energy bar be your vitality bite? Absolutely. But keep in mind that many of them are simply glorified candy bars. They can be high in protein but also high in sugar and fat, and most contain 200 to 250 calories. Convenience is the real draw. Easy to carry, easy to open, and easy to eat. But we might be just as well off with a cup of yogurt and some fruit.

Could a vitamin pill be your vitality bite? Not really. A vitamin pill has no calories, but sometimes a supplement can round out your diet and your energy level. What about those formulated specifically to "fight fatigue," "boost energy," "sustain stamina," and "enhance vitality"? They may outsmart your pocketbook a lot more than they outsmart your fatigue.

Fatigue Foolery: Don't Bite into the Hype

Maggie walked into my office for her first appointment with two bagfuls of her supplement intake—thirty-six different pills in all! She was spending over three hundred dollars a month but didn't feel that they were increasing her energy level. With fatigue now the number-one complaint from women, it's no surprise that Maggie and others turn to pills, potions, bars, and beverages that have been concocted to give us hope—and hype.

"But my doctor recommended all these. I buy them from him every month," Maggie argued, and my red flag went up. Any health professional who sells products often has profit as the underlying motive. According to the *Nutrition Business Journal*, over 350 million dollars' worth of wholesale vitamin products are sold to conventional and alternative medical practitioners—who in turn sell them for 700 million dollars. A 100 percent markup!

The claims made by the pill sellers or the pill manufacturers don't mean much—natural, high potency, time release, chelated, laboratory tested are all marketing terms. If you do take supplements, what's most important is to take them with meals and look for "USP" on the label. This stamp of approval tells you that the supplement meets high purity standards and has been tested to ensure that it dissolves in your stomach and is absorbed into your body. Tufts University did a study on non-USP pills and found that 40 percent did not dissolve. You can do your own test at home. Drop your supplement in a glass of vinegar and let it sit for thirty minutes. If, after this, the pill is still intact on the bottom of the glass, then it's not doing much good for your body.

Will herbs do your body good? Now that herbs have gone mainstream, the choices and claims are just as confusing as those for supplements. Ginseng is the herb most noted for its energizing properties. Although it has failed to hold up in most U.S. studies, there are some good European studies showing that it boosts stamina, endurance, and mood—but it doesn't work for everyone and may cause head-aches, depression, and insomnia in some. My research assistant and I did a little experiment with ginseng. We both took it for three days. She felt no boost; I felt a negative boost, more like nervous, hyper, unfocused energy. We all react differently to herbs. You may try it and like the short-term boost in energy, but I'll stick to caffeine for my morning jolt.

In addition to ginseng, other herbs are promoted for their ener-gizing or relaxing properties: garlic for physical energy, ginger for stamina, gotu kola for mental alertness, chamomile to calm the nerves, kava to relax the muscles, and valerian to reduce anxiety. These products won't harm you, but they may not help, either. One herb that may cause harm is ma huang (also known as ephedra), which boosts metabolism and acts like speed. A number of deaths have been associated with its use as a weight-loss aid and energy booster.

Most herbs and supplements won't harm you, but they won't give you the long-lasting vitality you're searching for, either. *Vitality comes from within—the connection of body, mind, and spirit that cre-ates a continuous flow of natural energy.* The 8 energizing strategies are your real secrets to maintaining this life-enhancing flow. And real food is one of them—the first and most important one. So instead of swallowing a pill, sink your teeth happily into satisfying, flavorful food—and give your mind, body, and spirit caloric energy!

HOW WILL YOU BEGIN SINKING YOUR TEETH INTO CALORIC ENERGY?

You have to do more than read about caloric energy—you have to start sinking your teeth into it every day! At the end of each strategy section, I'll ask you to specifically identify the techniques you'll use to outsmart your fatigue. Even if food deprivation is your biggest energy zapper, you don't have to follow everything recommended in this chapter, only what made sense for you and your lifestyle. If everything made sense, start slowly by choosing a half dozen techniques to practice for the next two weeks—then identify the next batch of vitality boosters you'll focus on.

So, how will you start sinking your teeth into vitality? Which eating-habit changes do you feel will give your energy the biggest boost? Using the following list, check all of the techniques you'll commit to for enhanced caloric energy.

_____ I will stop dieting, skipping meals, and restricting calories.

_____ I will fuel my body right away when I'm hungry.

_____ I will fill my stomach with a handful of food to prevent over-eating.

_____ I will eat smaller, more frequent meals.

_____ I will eat the majority of my small meals during the day and fewer at night.

_____ I will listen to my body and eat the foods I crave.

_____ I will eat a wide variety of foods, especially fruits and vegetables, to supply my body with the 8 energizing nutrients.

_____ I will eat foods high in carbohydrates every day.

_____ I will eat quality protein foods every day.

_____ I will eat some fat every day, especially monounsaturated fat.

_____ I will not eat sugar on an empty stomach.

_____ I will give pleasure to my taste buds with small bites of satisfying foods.

_____ I will smell my food before eating to stimulate my olfactory nerve.

_____ I will release food guilt and embrace eating pleasure.

_____ I will keep my list of "vitality bites" with me and eat these foods often.

_____ I will eat breakfast when my body is hungry and make sure it includes some carbohydrates and protein.

_____ I will take the time to eat a lunch that has sources of carbohydrates, protein, and fat.

_____ I will eat a small dinner that is mostly carbohydrates when I need to wind down or protein when I need to stay alert.

_____ I will snack throughout the day when my body is hungry.

_____ I will focus on food first and supplements second.

Chapter Four

WATER: TAKE A SIP OF HYDRAULIC ENERGY

No other substance is more abundant in all living things: Ninety percent of all plants are water, 60 percent of all animals are water, and 75 percent of the earth is water. No other element comprises more of the human body: Eighty-three percent of your blood is water, 75 percent of your brain is water, 70 percent of your muscle is water, and even 22 percent of your bone is water. No other nutrient is more essential for life: You can live without food for about five weeks, but you can live without water for only five days.

And no other fluid is more vital for energy. Water brings life-giving nutrients to your organs and cells and eliminates toxic waste products. It regulates body temperature and prevents heat exhaustion. It provides the medium for all biochemical reactions, including the formation of ATP energy molecules. When your body is dehydrated, you are devoid of energy. *Maybe today's lack of energy is due to yesterday's lack of water.*

Fatigue is the first and most common sign of dehydration. Your blood volume is decreased, your heart has to work harder to pump your reduced blood volume, your brain cells constrict, your head aches, you feel lightheaded, your muscle mass is in a drought, your legs feel like lead, and your cells can't produce ATP without H_2O. Dehydration negatively affects your ability to think, move, stand, exercise, sleep, work, make dinner, and make love. It even negatively affects your ability to lose weight. One study found that those who were just mildly dehydrated triggered their bodies' starvation response. They decreased their metabolism by 3 percent, stored more calories in their fat cells, and gained weight. Water could be your universal answer to outsmarting female fatigue *and* female fat cells.

Next to oxygen, water is the most necessary substance for life. You can live without bread alone (contrary to the popular saying), you can live without meat, you can live without fruits and vegetables (although not very well), you can even live without chocolate (well, at least some of us can)—but you can't live without water.

Although many of us try. The average woman consumes only two glasses of water a day, not nearly enough to replenish the loss of water through perspiration, respiration, urination, and defecation (FYI: Your stools are comprised of 40 percent water). For normal bodily functions alone, we need to replenish an average of two quarts a day, not two glasses.

Then there are other factors that cause greater water loss, greater dehydration, and a greater need to take a sip of hydraulic energy:

- If you exercise, your increased body temperature causes your cooling mechanism to kick in through sweating. Even if your sweats aren't drenched with sweat, water is still being rapidly evaporated through your skin. You can lose as much as two cups of water in an intense sixty-minute workout.

- If you live in a hot climate, the heat and humidity cause your sweat glands to work overtime, and you can lose up to an additional three cups a day.

- If you are in perimenopause or menopause, the hot flashes, night sweats, drenched sheets, and soaked clothes can dehydrate your body and trigger dizziness, headaches, heart palpitations, constipation, and lethargy.

- If you are the crying type who tears up when premenstrual, perimenopausal, just plain old sad, or watching a tear-jerking movie, the water loss can exceed that of a twenty-minute workout.

- If you take water-robbing drugs like diuretics, drink excessive amounts of coffee or tea, or consume alcoholic beverages, your water needs can increase substantially.

Add all of these together with the natural internal water losses, and most women walking around today are mildly to moderately dehydrated. Are you one of them?

This chapter will help assess your level of dehydration and determine how much water you need to drink to bring vitality back into your life. Your energy solution may be as simple as sipping more water. But how much should you sip? How often should you sip it? When should you sip? What kind of water should you sip? You may think that you know the answers to these questions, but today's popular water advice is overflowing with myths and misinformation.

GULP FICTION

Take this quiz to find out what you really know about water and optimal hydration. Answer each of the following statements as true or false.

	true	false
1. Drinking water before a meal will help you eat less.	_____	_____
2. Drinking water with your meal interferes with digestion.	_____	_____

	true	false
3. Drinking water cures acne.	___	___
4. Thirst is an accurate indicator of when to drink water.	___	___
5. If you don't sweat, than you don't have to drink as much water.	___	___
6. Coffee dehydrates your body.	___	___
7. Bottled water is better than tap water.	___	___
8. Mineral water provides significant minerals.	___	___
9. Water is the only beverage that will adequately hydrate your body.	___	___
10. Everyone needs eight glasses of water a day.	___	___

I had ten clients take this quiz, and every single one of them falsely thought each of the ten statements was true. Did you? Annmarie, who hates being wrong and never flunked a test in her life, was amazed that all of these were false and demanded an explanation to prove her wrong and dispel each of the myths. So here they are.

Drinking water before a meal does *not* help you eat less. Although it makes sense that a glass of water should fill you up and make you eat less food, the reality is that water is so quickly absorbed that your stomach is empty by the time you take your first bite. If you really want to eat less, drink a glass of fruit juice instead. A study in the *American Journal of Clinical Nutrition* reported that people ate less when the meal was preceded by juice—and ate more when it was preceded by water.

Drinking water with your meal does *not* interfere with digestion. This myth has been around for a while and for some reason continues to flourish. But the opposite is actually true. Because water is necessary for the breakdown of food and the absorption of nutrients, drinking water with your meal helps, rather than hinders, the digestive process. So keep that pitcher of water on your dinner table—and keep your glass full throughout the meal.

Drinking water does *not* cure acne. Although water is necessary for healthy skin overall, no study has proved that it's a solution for acne in adolescents or adults.

Thirst is *not* an accurate indicator of when to drink water. Thirst mechanisms are activated when you're already dehydrated. By then it's too late. You're fatigued, sluggish, and sleepy. To prevent dehydration and fatigue, you have to drink enough water to prevent your thirst mechanisms from even kicking into gear.

If you don't sweat, then you *do* have to drink as much water. Just because your sweat glands aren't active doesn't mean you don't actively have to pursue water. You may not have beads of sweat on your brow or water stains under your armpits, but you still evaporate water through your skin to cool your body—and you still need to drink plenty of water.

Coffee does *not* dehydrate your body. Unless you're drinking twelve or more cups per day, coffee doesn't put you in a negative water balance, as was previously thought. Caffeine is a diuretic, but a mild one. For every cup of coffee, you excrete one half of that cup through your urine. As a comparison, for every cup of water you drink, you excrete one third of it. Coffee may not dehydrate you, but it doesn't hydrate you as much as water, either. So to ensure proper hydration, make it a habit to chase your espresso with a glass of water.

Bottled water is *not* necessarily better than tap water. Twenty-five percent of all bottled waters are tapped from a municipal reservoir. So they can have the same potential contaminants and microorganisms as what comes out of your own tap. The remaining 75 percent of bottled water may or may not be better. It all depends on where they come from, how they are handled, and how they are tested. The United States' water supply, as we are repeatedly told, is the safest in the world, but many choose bottled water just to play it safe.

Mineral water does *not* supply significant minerals. Most contain such minuscule amounts that your local tap water may have more. A few European waters such as Perrier, Vittel, and San Pellegrino do have higher amounts of calcium, magnesium, and sodium—

but these amounts are not considered significant. You still have to eat your produce and drink your milk.

Water is *not* the only beverage that will adequately hydrate your body. It may be the best, but it's not the only one. Juice, milk, and electrolyte replacers such as Gatorade are also good hydrators. But soft drinks are too high in sugar content to provide an adequate water source for your body.

Everyone does *not* need eight glasses of water a day. Some people need five and others need twelve. In fact, there's very little research to support the eight-glass-a-day recommendation, except for those who live in a hot climate or engage in heavy physical exercise.

WHAT'S YOUR MAGIC NUMBER?

If your magic number isn't eight, what is it? On average, we need about two quarts of fluid to replace water loss. But the average is based on a man's body size and metabolism. Men's bodies have a higher water content than ours: 65 percent compared to our 50 percent. To bridge the gender gap between men and women where water is concerned, there are a number of ways you can determine how much water your female body needs to drink each day for optimal health and maximum energy.

1. **You can drink a cup for every 250 calories you eat.** For example, if you eat 1,750 calories a day, you need seven glasses of water. But to use this method, you have to count your calories daily, and I'd rather not have you caught up in that dieting numbers game.

2. **You can drink a cup for every twenty pounds you weigh.** So if you weigh 130 pounds, that's 6 and ½ cups. But to use this method, you have to use the bathroom scale on a regular basis, and I'd rather not have the scale become your measure of water bottles or self-worth.

3. **You can drink enough water to make your urine pale yellow in color.** If your urine is bright yellow and concentrated, keep

adding glasses until it's diluted and pale. This is my method of choice. And it's more accurate than the other two and just as accurate as a laboratory test. The only downside is that you may be spending more time in the bathroom with your eyes peeking in the toilet.

On different days, you may have different water needs depending on the outside temperature and humidity, how many hot flashes you've had, and your workout schedule—for each thirty-minute moderate-level workout, you need an additional cup of water. Your water needs are also dependent on whether you've consumed alcohol that day. Alcohol is a strong diuretic and puts your body in a negative water balance.

ALCOHOL, COFFEE, AND TEA: BOOST OR BUST?

Let's discuss alcohol first. Women are more prone to the effects of alcohol because of lower body weight, more body fat, less body water, and less alcohol dehydrogenase, the enzyme that breaks down and detoxifies alcohol. Therefore, we experience more of the dehydrating, depressing, and damaging effects of alcohol. We all know that alcohol is damaging to the liver, but is it dangerous for our breasts? That is a controversial and confusing question. Study results are across the board. Some show an increased risk for breast cancer with any amount of alcohol. Others reveal an increased risk only if we drink more than two glasses a day, or only if we're pre-menopausal, or only if we're postmenopausal. And still others show no increased risk at all. Pick your study—it's enough to drive you to drink!

But there has been some good news about booze. Many studies have shown that one or two drinks a day can reduce the risk of heart disease and stroke and increase longevity, especially when wine is our cocktail of choice. Danish researchers studied fifty thousand women and found that wine drinkers lived longer and had healthier diets than non-wine drinkers. They ate more fruits and vegetables and more fish and olive oil. Maybe it's not just the wine, but also the diet of wine drinkers that dictates how long and how well they live.

And then we have the French, who have often been sighted drinking wine with Brie, pâté, and croissants—and despite their high fat intake, they have one of the lowest risks of heart disease in the world. They drink ten times more wine than we do, but we seldom hear the flip side of their high alcohol consumption: that they also have twice the liver disease and cirrhosis that we do.

So before you run out for a jug of Chablis or a bottle of Opus One—think before you drink. Think moderate and think water. Alcohol of any kind is a powerful diuretic that increases urine output within a couple of hours, so drink a glass of water for every glass of wine or beer or hard liquor to prevent dehydration and post-alcohol fatigue. Or, you can do what my good friend Mary Pat does: Order your glass of chardonnay with a side of ice. After teasing her all these years about drinking her wine on the rocks, I have to commend her on her innovative hydrating strategy.

Now let's move on to coffee and tea. I've already discussed the myth that coffee is dehydrating; it's not—unless you drink quarts a day. But are coffee and other caffeinated beverages energizing? I'd have to answer "yes" and "no." Yes, because they activate your energy reserves, counteract sleepiness, raise blood pressure and heart rate, and increase concentration, alertness, attention span, productivity, and mood. And no, because the secondary effects of caffeine drain your energy reserves, make you sleepy, and decrease your concentration, alertness, attention span, productivity, and mood. You lose the energizing effects of caffeine within an hour or so—and then often turn to another cup to keep you going. Caffeine is a double-edged sword. It energizes you temporarily, fooling your body into thinking it has more energy. But eventually, your body realizes that it wasn't energized naturally and you become even more fatigued when the stimulating effects of the caffeine wear off. As one of my seminar attendees described it, you go from "caffeination elation" to "java the rut." It works in a pinch, but it doesn't work permanently, so then you're stuck in a fatigue rut. Perhaps the famous coffee slogan "good to the last drop" should read "good till you drop."

So now you know that in the long run, coffee is not dehydrating and not energizing. Now the question is: Is coffee safe to drink? The controversy on coffee continues to percolate.

Most researchers want to find something wrong with caffeine, but they just can't. Little, if any, evidence exists linking caffeine to benign breast lumps, kidney stones, cancer, hot flashes, and even osteoporosis. As long as you're getting enough calcium, caffeine appears to have no impact on fracture rates. Duke University Medical Center did find that more than four cups a day increased blood pressure and heart rate and prevented some people from falling asleep at night. (More on caffeine and insomnia in chapter 7.)

But let's define a cup. The "cup" all studies and recommendations refer to is a five-ounce teacup, not a coffee cup, travel cup, mug, Thermos, or grande at Starbucks. I don't know anyone who drinks coffee out of a teacup. Personally, I feel virtuous saying that I drink only one cup of coffee a day, but in all honesty, my mug has to hold at least twelve ounces. So if you're drinking two or three of these supersize mugs a day, you're way above a moderate level of one to two five-ounce cups a day and may be experiencing the negative effects of restlessness, rebound fatigue, stomach irritation, and insomnia.

Most of the research on coffee, however, has been neutral or even positive. The Harvard Nurses' Health Study showed that up to six cups a day produced no adverse effects on the female heart. Another highly publicized Harvard study discovered that caffeine positively influenced mood—so much so (presumably by increasing endorphins) that coffee drinkers had a 70 percent lower suicide rate than those who didn't drink it. And the University of California at Davis has always been nice to our vices. They first found antioxidents for us in wine, then in chocolate—and now they've found them in coffee. Antioxidents help to prevent heart disease and cancer, and the amount in a five-ounce cup of coffee adds up to three oranges!

But if it's antioxidents we're looking for, we'd be better off with a cup of tea. Green and black tea contain more powerful antioxidents than coffee. And after water, tea is the most popular beverage in the world. At least for everyone but us. We are grinders, not steepers. But many of us have started to replace our coffeepots with teapots. In the past five years, tea sales have quadrupled, and we're drinking 50 billion cups a year. Coffee still remains four times as popular, but tea is gaining ground, so to speak. If you're a tea drinker, keep two things in mind: 1) tea has less caffeine than coffee so it won't produce the lift you might be looking for, and 2) it's a stronger diuretic than coffee because of the chemical theophylline, which you may have already known because of more frequent visits to the bathroom. And less frequent visits to the dentist? Tea also contains fluoride, which inhibits tooth decay.

What about herbal teas? If they are caffeine-free, then they are also theophylline-free. But the herbs themselves may influence our energy and mood. The herbal tea aisle has grown in choice and in claims: Sleepy Time, Less Stress, Tension Tamer, Mood Mender, and High Energy are just a few of their packaging names. But a name is just a name, not a promise. However, there is some research to show that chamomile may act as a mild sedative, valerian may mimic a mild tranquilizer, ginger may calm the stomach, and peppermint may aid in breathing and bloatedness. Ever wonder why restaurants traditionally have a bowl of peppermint candies for the taking on the way out? To ease the bloated feeling from a hearty meal.

I was about to turn off my computer for a coffee break, but I think I'll have a cup of soothing tea instead.

SIPPING STRATEGIES TO STAY AFLOAT

After I shared all the benefits of water and hydration, my clever client Rachel said, "Well, you can lead a woman to water, but you can't make her drink." Because knowledge is one thing and behavior change another, here are some easy tips to encourage you to change your beverage behavior:

- Keep a glass of ice water on your desk while you're working—you'll be more inclined to take a sip every now and then.

- Keep a bottle of water with you while you're driving—and make red lights your green light to take a swig.

- Get a water cooler for your home, and lobby for one at your office.

- Start drinking a glass of water with every lunch or every dinner—or both.

- Pick a time of day (10 A.M., 2 P.M., 8 P.M.) that is designated water time—and commit to a cup every time the bell tolls.

These tips still didn't help Rachel because she claimed that she didn't like the taste of water. So I offered her these other options instead:

- Filter it—water filters can remove any off flavors that may turn your taste buds off as well as eliminate impurities that may concern you.

- Flavor it—add a slice of lemon, lime, or orange.

- Sparkle it—try tiny bubbles; some find the carbonation much more appealing.

- Experiment—try different bottled waters; you may discover that some taste better to you than others.

- Drink other beverages—juice is 90 percent water, milk is 87 percent water, and electrolyte drinks such as Gatorade are absorbed just as quickly as water.

And if all else fails—*eat your water.* Your food choices can add at least three cups of water a day, as long as you choose wisely.

Food	Water Content
watercress (hence the name)	95%
carrots	91%
most fruits and vegetables	80 to 90%
cottage cheese	80%
eggs	75%
potatoes and rice	70%
fish and shellfish	68%
pasta	65%
ice cream	60%
meats	55%
bread	35%
cheese	35%
dried fruit	20%
cereal and popcorn	5%

Rachel was most impressed with ice cream being 60 percent water, but the point is that you can hydrate your body to at least some extent with food as well as the faucet. If you eat five servings of fruits and vegetables a day, the recommendation from all major health organizations, that's the equivalent of two glasses of water right there. But a combination of water-packed foods and thirst-quenching beverages is most optimal for outsmarting your female fatigue.

There are some of us who think that if five or ten glasses of water keep our energy flowing, then fifteen or twenty will really open the fatigue-fighting floodgates. When something is good, more is not always better. Excess water acts as a diuretic and drains your energy as well as your bladder. You'll not only feel like you're drowning, you'll also feel like you could set up shop in the bathroom and take a nap right there. I recently had an ultrasound for which I had to drink eight glasses of water in thirty minutes . . . or else. I floated to the doctor's office, then wearily flushed the toilet at least a half dozen times over the next three hours.

THE WONDERS OF WATER WELLNESS

Water isn't just for drinking. It's for cleansing, swimming, playing, soaking, soothing, relaxing, and rejuvenating. Water is beneficial not only from the inside out, but also from the outside in.

Swimming in a mountain stream, diving in the ocean, soaking in the tub, standing beneath a shower of power, relaxing in a steam room, floating in a mineral bath—the name for these water pleasures is hydrotherapy, and you've used this type of therapy without consciously trying to: allowing the pounding pressure of the shower to energize you for a few minutes longer, lying in a bubble bath with no sense of time, or adding oils and fragrances to the tub for rejuvenating aromatic chemicals. Water *is* therapeutic, and Europeans have been privy to this little secret for centuries. From the ancient Roman bathhouses to the hot springs in Germany, hydrotherapy has been as fundamental to health as eating and sleeping. We've just begun to test the hydrotherapy waters, with spas popping up all over the country. Luckily, I live in northern California, where Napa Valley boils and bubbles with hot springs, mineral waters, and volcanic mud. My first introduction to hydrotherapy was almost twenty years ago in the famous mud baths of Calistoga. At first, I was a bit tentative about lying naked in a vat of bubbling mud, but when I had finished with the three-hour treatment of mud, tub, steam, massage, and mineral pools, I felt an energy surge that lasted for hours and had an afterglow that lasted for days.

So go ahead—play in the mud, dive in a lake, swim in a pool, soak in a tub, float in a mineral bath, relax in a Jacuzzi—and sip the refreshing, hydrating, energy-boosting beverage. ***Water really does work wonders.***

HOW WILL YOU BEGIN TAKING A SIP OF HYDRAULIC ENERGY?

Are you ready to hydrate your body and power your 75 trillion cells with cool, refreshing water? With the following list, check only those you feel will have the most impact on enhancing your hydraulic energy—and give yourself time to practice your chosen hydration boosters.

_____ I will drink enough water to make my urine pale in color.

_____ I will drink an additional glass of water for every cup of coffee or tea I consume.

_____ I will drink an additional glass of water for every alcoholic beverage I consume.

_____ I will drink an additional glass of water for every thirty-minute moderate-level workout.

_____ I will keep a glass of water on my desk while I'm working.

_____ I will keep a bottle of water with me while I'm driving my car or am in someone else's.

_____ I will drink a glass of water with every lunch.

_____ I will drink a glass of water with every dinner.

_____ I will pick a time of day (10 A.M., 2 P.M., 8 P.M.) that is designated water time.

_____ I will flavor my water with a slice of lemon, lime, or orange.

_____ I will try different bottled waters to see which one tastes best to me.

_____ I will consume other hydrating beverages such as milk, juice, and electrolyte drinks.

_____ I will "eat my water" by consuming more water-packed fruits and vegetables.

_____ I will use hydrotherapy to relax and rejuvenate my body.

Chapter Five

FITNESS: POWER YOUR BODY WITH PHYSICAL ENERGY

As much as some of us hate to admit it, we know that nothing energizes us more than exercise. It gets our hearts pumping, our lungs breathing, and our muscles contracting. It brings oxygen and nutrients to our cells, awakens our metabolism, alleviates a foul mood, and counteracts the negative effects of a bad-hair day. As much as we don't have the time or the energy to exercise after a hard day's work, we know that nothing will banish fatigue and silence stress more than a quick workout before dinner.

So why aren't we doing it? Despite the fitness boom of the 1980s and '90s, we're exercising *less* than we did a decade ago. Have the Jane Fondas, the Richard Simmonses, the Susan Powters, the Kathy Smiths, and the Denise Austins of the world gone unheard? I'm sure we've heard them (some of them are impossible to ignore); we just haven't heeded their advice to "work that body," "sweat to the oldies," "stop the insanity," or "jump on the fitness bandwagon." Or if we did jump on, we quickly jumped off after concluding that all that bouncing, gyrating, and pumping just wasn't for us.

Maybe aerobics classes, running, and weight lifting weren't for you, but the world of fitness has broadened in recent years to what I call a "no-pressure" approach that is easier on the body and kinder to the soul. You don't have to monitor your heart rate, go for the high-intensity burn, or pound the pavement for hours. All you have to do is move—and basically anything counts as exercise: weeding your garden, walking your dog, and even washing your car. If it's been years since you've attempted to pry your body off the couch, I encourage you to stand up and try again with the new information in this chapter. We all have reasons (excuses?) for why we don't exercise, but those reasons need to be reevaluated and updated for *no-pressure fitness*:

- **"I just don't like it."** You may not like exercise videos or pumping iron, but would you find ballet or beach walking more enjoyable? Or how about yoga or swing dancing?

- **"It's boring."** I find many exercises boring, too. Peddling on a stationary bike going nowhere is not my idea of a good time, but playing golf or hiking in the mountains is stimulating and invigorating.

- **"I don't have the time."** There are 336 half hours in one week; couldn't you spare a couple of them? The time it takes to revitalize your body through fitness is a fraction of what you've been told in the past. It no longer takes hours; it only takes minutes. In fact, ten minutes is often enough to recharge your energy.

- **"I don't like to sweat."** You don't have to. A ten-minute walk won't leave you drenched and a quick run up a flight of stairs won't require a change of clothes.

- **"I'm too out of shape to exercise."** You're too out of shape *not* to exercise. An out-of-shape body tires more easily and can lead to out-of-this-world fatigue. Start slowly and gradually build your level of fitness. The more fit you become, the more energy you'll have to exercise.

- **"I'm embarrassed to exercise because I'm too fat."** We think the whole world is watching us and making disparaging comments, but the reality is that the world has more important things to worry about than your body. Do it for *you*—and do it in the privacy of your home if that makes you feel more comfortable.

- **"My breasts will droop from all that bouncing."** You don't have to bounce at all; you can glide through the water or stroll in the park. But wearing a supportive bra is a good idea anyway.

- **"I'll become the 'incredible bulk.' "** You won't bulk up unless you're bench-pressing 150 pounds. Fit muscles are smaller in size than unfit muscles—and fit people are smaller in size than unfit people.

- **"I don't like pain."** As Lydia said, "If I wanted to inflict pain, I'd get back with my ex-husband before I started exercising." The "no pain, no gain" slogan was a product of the stressed-out, push-yourself-to-the-limit twentieth century. With a new century and a new approach to fitness, exercise needn't cause any pain; in fact, it should help ease pain—from back problems, arthritis, fibromyalgia, carpal tunnel syndrome, and migraines, as well as from emotional stress, traumatic past experiences, and irritating ex-husbands.

- **"I don't need to exercise; I was born fit."** My client Kathy read somewhere that some people were born with a "fit" gene. They maintain their weight, energy, muscle strength, and metabolism without ever lifting a limb. If we could all be so lucky. But 99.9 percent of us aren't, so if you're feeling tired and worn out, you weren't born with this gene. You can still, however, initiate your energy rebirth through ***no-pressure fitness.***

My favorite exercise excuse is from a client who told me, "I tried jogging once but had to give it up for my health. My thighs kept rubbing together and setting my shorts on fire." If we're not going to exercise, we might as well have a sense of humor about it.

Do you have an outdated exercise excuse that's preventing you from using no-pressure fitness to power your body? Do you avoid exercise at all costs, or do you take the opportunity to move whenever you can? Have you started and stopped exercising a dozen times, or have you started exercising and haven't stopped moving since you took your first Jazzercise class?

There are basically four types of exercisers:

1. **Non-exercisers.** At least 30 percent of us do absolutely nothing—nada, zip, zero, zilch. We may be adamant exercise haters or simply be waiting for someone to come up with a routine for recliner aerobics.

2. **Occasional exercisers.** Thirty to 40 percent of us dabble in intermittent bouts of exercise. We might play tennis once a week, play golf once a month, go bowling once in a while, ride our bikes now and then, or join a new gym every January only to cancel our membership by March.

3. **Regular exercisers.** Only 20 percent of us are motivated movers. We go to a health club at lunchtime, meet friends for a sunrise walk, ride the stationary bike at night, or make sure we don't miss our weekend spinning class.

4. **Excessive exercisers.** An estimated 10 to 20 percent of us have entered the exercise danger zone. We're trying to exercise almost every day for hours at a time, thinking that more exercise will defy Mother Nature; counteract the effects of gravity; preserve a thin, youthful body, and turn back Father Time. But no amount of exercise can accomplish these feats—and *too much exercise can be just as tiring as too little.*

Which category do you fall into? If you're a regular exerciser, you could probably skip this chapter because you know the pleasures of powering your body with physical energy. But nevertheless, I encourage you to continue reading to discover new, energizing ways to tailor your exercise program for lifelong vitality.

If you're an occasional exerciser, you'll be pleased to hear that you may be doing enough or almost enough to outsmart your female fatigue. Even occasional bouts of exercise fuel your energy. If you're moving your body weekly or a few times a month, I still suggest at least skimming the following pages for new ways you can maximize your energy with minimal additional effort.

Now, if you're a non-exerciser or an excessive exerciser, I recommend neither skipping nor skimming, but carefully studying this chapter. It was written for *you*. With either extreme of exercise, you're not using fitness to fight fatigue. Therefore, my overriding goal is to motivate those of you who do nothing to do something— and to encourage those who do too much to do less.

"Do less?" the excessive exercisers gasp. "I've spent years building my muscle mass and reducing my body fat. I can't do less than six days a week for one hundred twenty minutes a day." "Do something!" the non-exercisers protest. "Not if it involves sweating, showering, changing my clothes, and huffing and puffing like an animal in heat every day."

To silence your protests, let's start with the good news: You don't have to exercise every day for it to have a positive influence on your level of energy. *Even once a week will help your energy reach its peak. Even ten minutes will jump-start your stamina*—without a change of clothes. To maximize your vitality through fitness, however, three to five times a week for thirty-plus minutes is recommended. But we'll talk about that later. First, I just want to help you non-exercisers do something!

It doesn't matter if you consider yourself the "queen of couch potatoes" or the president of the I-Hate-Exercise club. It doesn't matter if you haven't moved a muscle since high school gym class or haven't walked a mile since your car ran out of gas six years ago. You can still worship your couch, refuse to join a gym, ban leotards from your home, and leave the exercise equipment in the garage collecting cobwebs. The *only* prerequisite is that you have to do something. Anything. And I guarantee that you'll experience the energizing benefits of fitness.

RIDE THE MOOD ELEVATOR

When you're feeling low, wouldn't it be great if you could jump on a platform, push a button, and bring your energy level up a couple of notches? As you know, it's not quite that easy, but exercise can quickly transport you to a higher energy state. If you went out for a ten-minute brisk walk right now, you'd increase blood flow, oxygen delivery, and ATP formation—and would feel a boost in energy that would last for up to two hours! One hundred and twenty minutes of stamina for a ten-minute investment. Not a bad return. Why don't you try it right now? If your fatigue is telling you to go out for a ten-minute wonder walk, then take a break and hitch a ride on the mood elevator. You'll come back ready and raring to go for the next few hours.

If, instead of stopping after ten minutes, you gradually increased your walking time to thirty minutes every other day, you'd experience the long-term vitality benefits of fitness. Your heart would grow stronger and larger, you'd more efficiently deliver nutrients and oxygen to your cells, and you'd develop more capillaries to increase blood supply to your brain, muscles, and all your internal organs. You'd feel better, improve your overall level of fitness, and increase your daily energy. Studies have shown that regular, consistent movement at least three times a week for thirty minutes adds 25 percent more energy to every waking moment. And if you did this for the rest of your life, you'd maintain muscle strength, metabolism, mobility, agility, and vitality—even through your ninth decade. It's true. Fit ninety-year-olds have more energy than most less fit sixty-year-olds. Think of the fit energetic elders in your life. Did they belong to a health club? No. Did they take heart-pounding aerobics classes? No. They simply moved their bodies on a regular basis by gardening, kneading bread, scrubbing the floors, hand-washing their clothes, and walking to the store—thereby maintaining their youthful vitality.

Not only does exercise give you an immediate boost, a long term energy supply, and lifelong vitality, it also generally improves your mood. Having time alone away from the screaming kids, the barking dog, the demanding boss, and the soliciting phone calls is uplifting by itself. But exercise also brightens your mood through these powerful physiological changes:

- **It increases serotonin and the endorphins**—and these "feel good" brain chemicals will keep you smiling, with a more positive outlook on life.

- **It increases body temperature**—a higher than normal body temperature can have a tranquilizing effect, calming you during your most stressful times.

- **It reduces anxiety**—as long as you don't bring your frustrations to the workout room. An interesting study was done on college students during finals week. When they leisurely rode a stationary bike for twenty minutes, they reduced their anxiety level by 50 percent. But when they studied their textbooks while pedaling, their anxiety level stayed high.

- **It reduces depression**—the positive effect of exercise on depression has been reported in over 100 scientific papers. Not only does it help those who are clinically depressed, but it also aids those who periodically feel blue.

If these energy-boosting, mood-altering benefits didn't eject you out of your chair for a ten-minute wonder walk, then consider these other extended health benefits. In addition to riding the mood elevator, fitness will also help you to:

- **Jog your memory**—fit sixty-year-olds have better short-term memories than unfit thirty-year-olds. Exercise prevents your brain from shrinking and your memory from getting misplaced as you grow older.

- **Stretch your imagination**—here's a fascinating study: Middlesex University in England took two groups of people and had one group sit still while the other participated in a twenty-five-minute aerobics class. The two groups were then put in separate rooms and given the assignment to come up with innovative ways to use tin cans. The sitters could come up with only the obvious vase or pencil holder, but the exercisers used their imagination to build rockets and decorative Christmas ornaments.

• **Race for the cure**—the University of Southern California School of Medicine found that regular exercisers reduced their risk of breast cancer by 30 percent. Another study on 73,000 women found that as activity level went up, heart disease risk went down. *Fitness fights disease.*

• **Build your bone bank**—Tufts University found that a one-year walking program increased bone density by 1 percent, whereas those who were sedentary continued to lose 1 percent per year. *Exercise not only prevents bone loss but promotes bone growth.*

• **Climb into bed**—the University of Arizona found that those who exercised just once a week had 38 percent fewer sleep disturbances than those who didn't exercise.

• **Walk away from weight gain**—the only way to take weight off and keep it off is through a regular exercise program. I could share hundreds of studies, but the most convincing evidence comes from your own community. Look around you. Those you see walking down the street or working in their gardens are leaner. Those who sit around stay round.

• **Run for your life**—the University of Minnesota School of Public Health followed forty thousand women and found that those who exercised just once a week were 24 percent less likely to die prematurely than those who didn't exercise at all.

If a longer life, better memory, heightened creativity, stronger bones, healthier breasts, a leaner body, more energy, heightened mood, and sounder sleep don't motivate you—then how about . . . better sex? With exercise, you'll also feel the earth move. Fit women (and fit men for that matter) report a more satisfying sex life.

To experience all of these mental and physical benefits, exercising just once a week for ten to thirty minutes is enough to start doing your body good. Could you exercise once in the next seven days for ten minutes? Most say, "Well, sure." Others say, "If once a week gives me better sex, more energy, and a leaner body—then every day will give me great sex, maximum energy, and an ultra-skinny body." Unfortunately, fitness doesn't work that way. *Exercise powers your body, but too much can leave you powerless.*

FITNESS FATIGUE: TOO MUCH OF A GOOD THING

Just last week, I saw three new clients who were overtired because they were overtiring their bodies with too much exercise. One woman was running twice a day, another was spending three hours at her health club taking back-to-back step classes, and the third was an aerobics instructor teaching four classes a day. All three were perplexed when I told them that in order to increase their energy, they needed to decrease their activity.

Exercise has an amazing effect on raising your energy—up to a point, then it starts to rob you of energy. The irony of fitness is that it takes energy to make energy. To contract your muscles and move your body, you use ATP energy molecules, calories, and oxygen. But the end result is that you'll make *more* ATP, rev up your metabolism, and boost your stamina for hours after you exercise. Up to four hours of exercise a week and you'll feel a noticeable energy return on your investment. At five and six hours a week, your energy gain plateaus, and at seven hours you'll start to feel an energy loss. After eight hours, you'd almost have more energy if you didn't exercise at all.

Let me explain the strange phenomenon of fitness fatigue. Overexercise makes you overtired by:

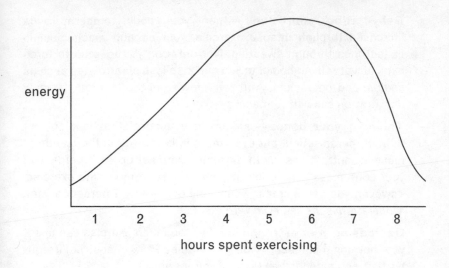

energy

1   2   3   4   5   6   7   8

hours spent exercising

- **Depleting your glycogen stores**—after one hour of nonstop exercise, your body stops burning primarily fat and starts to rely on glycogen stores in your muscles and liver to keep you moving. When these stores are diminished, you feel weak and lethargic. When the stores are gone, you "hit the wall," a phrase used by the running world that means you absolutely cannot take another step.

- **Dropping your metabolism**—overexercise is like dieting. You're burning too many calories through exercise, and your body feels threatened. So it goes into starvation mode to conserve calories and enhance your survival. Take female marathon runners as an example. Studies have shown that many need only 1,400 calories a day to maintain their weight while the typical active woman needs about 2,000. You'd think the marathon runners' hunger would force them to wolf down over 3,000 calories a day, but their overtraining undermines their metabolism.

- **Stressing your bones and joints**—sports medicine clinics are making more money than ever by treating stress fractures, torn ligaments, and knee problems. Most sports-related injuries are caused by too much exercise and not enough rest.

- **Dehydrating your body**—when your body temperature is increased through intense exercise, your cooling mechanism is called upon through sweating. Not only can you lose up to three cups of water in an hour, but you can also lose electrolytes such as sodium and potassium. And you know from the last chapter how dehydration can wilt your energy.

- **Thinning your bones**—calcium is a mineral that is also lost through perspiration, but even more is lost through thousands of muscle contractions. With extreme exercise, up to 3 percent of your bone mass can be lost in one year. With moderate exercise, however, you can increase your bone density by 1 percent a year. *Moderation is the key, even with exercise.*

- **Decreasing your estrogen levels**—too much exercise can upset your hormonal balance, leading to intense PMS, menstrual irregularities, and amenorrhea (loss of your periods).

- **Compromising your immune system**—those running sixty miles a week while training for the Los Angeles Marathon had twice the colds and flus as those running a more recreational twenty miles a week.

- **Increasing your risk of death**—not from a heart attack or rottweiler attack, but, in the long run, from the body-wearing effects of overexercise. Studies at Stanford University and the Cooper Institute in Dallas found that exercise reduces death rates until we start overexercising. More than eight hours a week and death rates start to climb.

Exercise will *not* be energizing if it kills you, makes you sick, causes injury, or wears you out. Are you overexercising?

Most of the overexercisers I know do not consider themselves overexercisers. They call themselves "devout runners," "health club groupies," or "fitness divas" and think they need to keep doing more, not start doing less. Their drive to overexercise is often due to their drive for thinness. Fitness is used more as a weapon against the battle of the bulge than for the fight against fatigue, and they attack exercise with the same compulsive behavior that they used with dieting—quick weight loss, going for the "burn," getting on the scale, and using weight loss as a distraction from other problems in their lives that need to be addressed. Maybe we need to pay less attention to our abs and more to our lives. Maybe we need to stop spending so much time shaping our thighs and start shaping our lives. Unlike compulsive dieting, eating, drinking, or gambling, compulsive exercising is almost considered to be a virtuous sign of willpower and self-discipline. It's not. It's a sign of self-destruction and is an unhealthy behavior.

Ask any serious athlete about the negative effects of overexercising. She (or he) will tell you about potential problems of having fitness take over your life and eventually lead to exercise exhaustion. She'll also share with you the solution to fitness fatigue: Take at least one to two days off a week to replenish glycogen, repair muscle, and strengthen your body. *Adequate rest is just as important as regular movement.*

If you're overexercising, I encourage you to do an experiment for a month and limit your workouts to no more than five times a week for an hour each. Note how your strength and energy reappear—but your body fat doesn't. If you're a non-exerciser, you may find this section a bit irrelevant: How can you overexercise when you're not exercising? Use the information in this chapter to prevent any possibility of overexercising in the future and try a different experiment: For the next month, consider exercising one to three times a week for ten to thirty minutes and see how it feels to power your body with physical energy.

EXERCISE YOUR OPTIONS

The choice to exercise is yours and yours alone. No one can force you to start exercising. You have to pick, choose, prioritize, and self-prescribe exercise. And your options are endless.

You can go the traditional route with a health club membership or a walking routine. Or you can do something completely different that doesn't feel like exercise at all. You can:

- Take a self-defense class—maybe you've always wanted to.

- Learn the samba or the tango—or try Flamenco dancing or belly dancing.

- Take golf lessons—perhaps you have a gift certificate somewhere that you got for your birthday two years ago.

- Try the more meditative movements like yoga, tai chi, and Pilates—these exercises are thousands of years old and are backed up by evidence that proves they increase circulation, strength, and stamina.

- Take an innovative aerobics class—some of the new ones include gospel moves where you dance to choir music and firefighter fitness taught by real firemen. Now that sounds like fun!

- Go bowling—a typical bowler lifts a thousand pounds in a three-game series.

- Check out this list of unusual options that can energize you more than standard exercise movements:

Ping-Pong	can be more energizing than	walking
square dancing	"	riding a bike
mowing the lawn	"	an aerobics class
raking leaves	"	weight lifting
gardening	"	aqua aerobics
horseback riding	"	strength training
food shopping	"	playing Frisbee
running up stairs	"	cross-country skiing

Another option is to take something you already do and modify it to make it your designated energy exercise time:

- When you vacuum, move faster and push the vacuum harder. Envision yourself vacuuming away your fatigue.

- When you take the dog out to do his business, walk briskly around the block while you're at it.

- When you go to the grocery store, park at the end of the lot, move the cart faster, and carry your own groceries out.

- When you go to the department store, take the stairs to the upper floors instead of the elevator or escalator.

- If you play a musical instrument, play it more often and for longer periods of time. Playing most instruments burns at least 160 calories an hour.

When you do these and other common activities, do them for at least ten minutes and with the purpose of boosting your energy. And if none of these options interests you, you can always fidget. People who fidget energize their bodies by burning up to an extra seven hundred calories a day (but you have to be a serious fidgeter to burn that many). The University of Vermont found that people who squirm in their seats, tap their feet, play with their hair, and can't sit still had bodies that were resistant to weight gain even when they overate. The scientific term for fidgeting is "non-exercise activity thermogenesis." In other words, activities that burn calories and produce heat ("thermo" means heat and "genesis" means formation) without formally exercising.

Some people are natural-born fidgeters. Ever since childhood, they haven't been able to keep still. Do you know any? What's their body weight? What's their energy level? If you aren't a natural-born fidgeter, mimic their behavior and consciously train yourself to fidget by:

- standing while you talk on the phone

- putting on music and dancing while you're doing the dishes

- talking with your hands (easier for those from certain ethnic backgrounds to do than for others)

- changing your position, recrossing your legs, and sitting forward

- setting a timer for every thirty minutes and tapping your feet thirty times

And you'll be exercising without really exercising!

While you're exercising your exercise options, also exercise patience, perseverance, and persistence. Persistence is a desirable trait that leads to success in anything you do. Thomas Edison is famous for saying that "genius is 1 percent inspiration and 99 percent perspiration." If at first you don't succeed in fitness, try, try again. There is an activity out there that's right for you!

REVIVAL OF THE FITTEST

Any exercise will unlock your physical power and help you find the vitality within you. *Every* movement will help you outsmart your female fatigue. *Every woman* has an energetic, fit person inside her that's just waiting to get out. Even one of my best pals, Joyce, has one, although she denied it at first by joking, "If I do have a fit person inside me somewhere, she can usually be quickly sedated with a bag of tortilla chips and guacamole."

Let me tell you about Joyce. For years, the mere mention of the "e" word brought a "don't even start" look that immediately shut me up. But I'd always manage to say, "When you're ready, I'm ready. Just say the word." One day about eight months ago, we were together for one of our marathon catch-up-on-life sessions when she said, "Okay, I'm ready." I thought she was ready for another glass of wine, so I started pouring. "No," she clarified, "I'm ready to start exercising." And that was it. We talked for hours about her needs and wants, set her up with a personal trainer to get her started, and then she was off and walking—four times a week for forty-five minutes each time. It's been great fun to watch her become a fit person who has a constant glow of energy, a happy bounce in her step, and a reshaped pair of legs that go up to her neck and could stop traffic.

If Joyce can let her fit person out, you can, too. She's there. Find her and revive her by keeping these ten tips in mind:

1. **Do _only_ what you like.** If walking in place on a treadmill doesn't turn you on, then don't do it. If dancing to old disco tunes does, then so be it.

2. **Make it fun.** Think back to the days when you used to hop on your Schwinn, swing in the park, and play hide-and-seek in your backyard. Fitness can and should still be fun in adulthood.

3. **Think of your exercise as a "time out" from daily stressors.** Don't carry your cell phone or pager with you while you exercise, although many do. Instead, drown out any distracting noises by listening to Mozart on your Walkman.

4. **Schedule it in.** Take out your day planner and write in your ten-minute wonder walks. Today at 4:15 P.M.? Tomorrow at 10:30 A.M.? Don't let them be the first thing you cross off when you get behind schedule; cross something else off instead.

5. **Combine short-term bursts with longer boosts.** Use your ten-minute activities for a burst of energy any time of the day or night, and, for the long run, use your thirty-plus-minute exercises to keep fatigue away.

6. **Find the right time.** Although late afternoon may seem to be the best time to energize your body because you're the most fatigued, do it whenever it's best for you and your schedule. Any time of day is the right time to exercise.

7. **Find a fitness partner.** Those who walk with a friend or a group are more likely to still be strolling for stamina ten years later. Even if you don't feel like exercising, you're more likely to force yourself to do it when you know your partner is waiting for you at the park or the gym.

8. **Drink before you move.** A glass of water thirty minutes before a workout will prevent dehydration fatigue.

9. **Don't call it exercise.** Call it your metabolism booster, your energy break, your ten-minute wonder walk, your tension time-out, or the activity formally known as exercise.

10. **Help a friend.** When a friend tells you that she's lost her energy, tell her you know exactly where it is and can help her find it. "It's

just down the block, around the corner, and to the left." And, no, she can't drive there, she has to walk.

SO WHERE'S YOUR GYM BAG?

As a Chinese proverb tells us, "A journey of a thousand miles begins with a single step." Your first step may be finding your gym bag that's buried in the closet, buying a good pair of walking shoes, deciding what exercise option you'll choose, and/or picking a start date. It could be tomorrow, next week, or next month. Remember: This is **no-pressure fitness**. But the sooner you start, the sooner you'll feel energized.

I've tried to approach exercise differently in this book than in my other books. Instead of exercising to burn fat, get lean, prevent disease, or live longer, I've encouraged exercise to connect you to your physical power, strength, and stamina. Not a means to an end, but an end in and of itself.

Maybe we should call it *innercise* instead of exercise. Movement that ignites energy from within. Fitness that powers your body by putting you in touch with your internal fire. When you make fitness a part of your life, something seems to click internally, and other areas of your life begin to change for the better. People who exercise are more likely to drink adequate water, eat five small meals a day, sleep more restfully, get more sunshine and fresh air, have more intimate friendships, foster a better body image, and have a happier, less stressed outlook on life.

You may recognize these added benefits of "innercise"—they are the 8 energizing strategies to lifelong vitality. Maybe all we need to do is start moving our bodies and we'll automatically start outsmarting our female fatigue in every possible way. Welcome fitness into your life and see for yourself.

HOW WILL YOU BEGIN POWERING YOUR BODY WITH PHYSICAL ENERGY?

Are you exercising too little or too much? How will you change your exercise attitude and fitness behavior to revitalize your body with physical energy? With the following list, check all that you'll commit to for inner strength, power, and stamina.

_____ I will remind myself of all the benefits of exercise and think "no-pressure fitness."

_____ I will confront my past exercise excuses and approach fitness with a fresh attitude.

_____ I will start exercising a minimum of once a week for ten minutes.

_____ I will build my exercise program to three to five times a week for thirty-plus minutes.

_____ I will not push my body too hard or exercise more than eight hours a week.

_____ I will move my body with nontraditional exercises such as dance, golfing, yoga, tai chi, bowling, gardening, and horseback riding.

_____ I will take an activity I already do (such as walking the dog or cleaning the house) and do it with the purpose of boosting energy.

_____ I will fidget more in the standing and sitting positions.

_____ I will find an activity I like and the time of day that's best for me to do it.

_____ I will schedule my ten-minute wonder walks in my day planner.

_____ I will find a fitness partner to keep me motivated.

_____ I will drink a glass of water thirty minutes before my workout to prevent dehydration.

_____ I will pick a start date to welcome fitness into my life.

_____ I will think "innercise" instead of "exercise."

Chapter Six

THE GREAT OUTDOORS: SURROUND YOURSELF WITH NATURAL ENERGY

As I begin writing this chapter, I find myself in a most opportune location—on the northern California coast, a place called The Sea Ranch, or as the residents and visitors refer to it: God's Country. With over 100 miles of hiking trails, the Pacific Ocean in your vision, the redwood mountains at your back, whales migrating, seals barking, deer roaming, and numerous species of birds chirping, you can't help but feel and respond to the powerful force of nature.

I seek out this place often, for rest, relaxation, solitude, peace, rejuvenation, and inspiration. It comes as no surprise that I do my best writing here. Whether I'm at the desk gazing out at the wildflowers and trees, on the deck periodically looking up at the blowing wheat fields and crashing waves, or on the beach with notebook in hand and sand on my feet, I'm surrounded by natural energy, effortlessly taking it in and letting it stimulate my mind and body.

Do you have a special spot where you're surrounded by the sights, sounds, and smells of nature? Maybe you're lucky enough to live in such a place, or grew up there before you took off for the big city. Perhaps you escape to a special haven for weekend retreats or pack up and go camping, boating, backpacking, hiking, or mountain climbing for weeks at a time. Even if you're not the "outdoor type," when you're surrounded by natural energy, it's almost impossible not to also power your body with physical energy via nature walks, berry picking, seashell collecting, or other simple outdoor activities. Whether you have daily experience with Mother Nature's rejuvenating magic or haven't felt her force since your childhood days of summer camp, this chapter will encourage you to take full advantage of her fresh air, bright sunshine, aromatic flowers and plants, colorful landscapes, breathtaking vistas, hiking trails, sandy beaches, clear lakes, and babbling brooks. Tapping into nature's energy source may be the easiest strategy of all. It requires minimal effort and is right there for the taking. All you have to do is open your door to the great outdoors and let Mother Nature beckon you.

AND NOW, A WORD FROM MOTHER NATURE

How much time do you spend outdoors every day? "I have an attached garage so I don't leave the house in the morning. Then I park my car in the lot under my office building, take the elevator straight up to the sixteenth floor, work in a cubicle all day, eat lunch in the building cafeteria, and most of the time go straight home after work. At least three days a week, I never see the light of day."

No wonder Maria was so tired. No sun, no fresh air, no visual stimulation. But Maria's nature void is not all that unusual; on average, we spend 95 percent of our time indoors, and much of our outdoor time is between the car and our next indoor destination. When was the last time you walked to a park for an afternoon break? Ate lunch at an outdoor café? Drove to the beach for a swim? Sat outside to drink your morning coffee? Flew a kite on a Sunday afternoon? Stepped outdoors to view the blooming flowers? If Mother Nature could talk to us, she'd gently encourage us to surround ourselves with her natural energy by saying, "Just step outside for a moment and see my vibrant colors, smell my sweet aromas, hear my calming sounds, and feel my cool breezes."

Nature quickly restores our energy and outsmarts our fatigue because it is pleasing to all five of our senses.

1. **Sight.** Viewing the spectacular colors of sunrise and sunset, a rainbow on the horizon, flowers blooming in spring, the leaves changing color in autumn, or the first pure white snow of winter can stimulate the visual center in your brain. If you have tired eyes from computer work and paperwork, nature's sights can soothe your eyes and clear your mind.

2. **Smell.** The fragrant scents of flowers, the woody air of a forest, and the salty breeze of the ocean can ignite your olfactory nerve and awaken your brain.

3. **Hearing.** The sounds of birds chirping, waves crashing, rain falling, and leaves rustling in the wind can calm your stress with rhythmic, melodic tones.

4. **Touch.** The soft drizzle of rain on your face, the cool breeze in your hair, and the warmth of sunshine on your body can stimulate your skin's touch receptors and renew your spirit.

5. **Taste.** Fresh seasonal fruit, homegrown tomatoes, and vegetables from the farmer's market can give pleasure to your taste buds and satisfy your brain. Before food processors, convection ovens, microwaves, canned goods, and frozen foods, we relied on nature's abundant supply of plants, trees, seeds, spices, herbs, and flowers for nourishment. Ever since Euell Gibbons's famous line in the 1970s, "Have you ever eaten a tree? Many parts *are* edible," we've been urged to get back to nature with our eating. Despite the fact that he didn't live long enough to witness his sage advice take hold, more and more people have realized that wholesome, natural food gives their bodies natural, caloric energy.

Your five senses are eagerly waiting to be stimulated by nature and your sixth sense—intuition—is encouraging you to take full advantage of the great outdoors. Instinctively, you've always known that the sun's rays, the moon's pull, the flower's fragrance, and the fresh air affect the way you feel. In fact, studies have shown that women are more in tune with all six senses than men. We have better hearing, keener smell, and more touch receptors on our skin for reasons of survival and childbearing. In order to hear the cries of distress at night, to feel the touch of a child's needy hand, or to smell the scent of impending danger, our bodies react more quickly by recognizing the stimulus and responding immediately. Some interesting research has been done on the gender differences in smell, and especially around ovulation, we are ten thousand times more sensitive to certain smells, including smoke, wild animals, and men. Not that men are necessarily a sign of danger, but we are drawn to the smell of their male pheromones during the fertile times of our cycle.

So let's use our biologically advanced sensory system to reap the benefits of Mother Nature. You can choose a simple activity such as planting a rock garden, watching a sunset, or swimming in a lake. Or you can do something on a grander scale like landscaping your yard, scuba diving in the ocean, or visiting the desert, mountains, or a national park. Whatever you do to surround yourself with natural energy, do it with intent, focus, and concentration—or, as the New Agers would say, do it *mindfully*.

I am reminded of Chevy Chase in the movie *National Lampoon's Vacation* when he stops the car at the Grand Canyon, gets out, and immediately says, "Okay. Let's go." Even when we see nature at its finest, we're often too rushed to really see it, connect with it, and take it all in. Sometimes we ride by it on a bus tour, or we're too busy videotaping it to truly experience it, or we're too preoccupied with where we need to go next to appreciate where we are right now.

Where are you right now? If you're someplace where you can step outside and into the wonder of Mother Nature, do it and get lost in her sights, sounds, and scents for a few minutes. You'll come back refreshed and ready to finish the rest of this chapter.

REJUVENATE YOUR SOUL WITH SOLAR ENERGY

Let me shed some light on the subject of fatigue. Sunlight is one of nature's most powerful energy sources. If solar energy can heat your home and your pool, it can also heat up your vitality, give you a sunny disposition, and brighten your mood. The sun's rays have been found to release brain serotonin, reduce stress, nourish your body with vitamin D, synchronize your body's rhythms, and calm PMS and menopausal tension. A study at the University of California at San Diego found that bright-light exposure one week before women started their periods significantly reduced many premenstrual symptoms, including depression and fatigue—thus *proving that there is light at the end of the PMS tunnel!*

When our bodies are deprived of sunshine, we're deprived of energy, health, and happiness. Anytime we purposely avoid the sun, we miss out on an important energy source and, as a result, experience greater daytime fatigue. And whenever winter approaches, the shorter daylight hours can cause lethargy, sleepiness, moodiness, and the "winter blues." The extreme effect of winter darkness is called Seasonal Affective Disorder (with the appropriate acronym SAD), in which months of ongoing sun deprivation negatively interfere with your work, family, and social life.

Seasonal changes in energy level, mood, and sleeping behavior are strongly tied to day length. How do you feel in October as the days become shorter and we move the clocks back an hour? How do you feel in February after five months of shorter days and cloudy skies? What happens in April when you experience your spring awakening? And how about July when the days are long and the sun is strong?

Of course, how much you're affected by the change of seasons has to do with where you live. Your latitude affects your attitude, so to speak. The Pacific Northwest has the highest incidence of SAD; the South has the lowest. But even southern Californians, Texans, and Floridians feel the effects of shorter days on their biological rhythms and sleep/wake cycles. If you do, regardless of where you live, there is much you can do to light up your life and extinguish your fatigue:

- **Step outside as soon as you wake up.** Early morning light synchronizes your body's rhythms for the rest of the day.

- **Use high noon sun to heighten your energy.** The sun's rays are the brightest then and will cause your brain to release the most serotonin.

- **Sit near a window whenever you can.** Your brain will recognize that it's still daytime and will keep you awake.

- **Install a skylight or two.** This will provide some additional light even when the sun is starting to set.

- **Move to a southern state.** An extreme option, but many have relocated to relieve their winter blues.

- **Go south for a winter break.** Spending a week's vacation in Florida, the Caribbean, Mexico, or Hawaii may be a more feasible option and is a frequent recommendation by SAD experts.

- **Try light therapy.** Instead of spending a couple of thousand dollars on an island holiday, spend a couple of hundred dollars on a light box.

Designed to sit on your desk or table, light boxes mimic the intensity of the sun's rays, measured by the number of lux (lux is a measurement of the intensity or brightness of light). A typical light-bulb has only 500 lux of light intensity, but a light box has 2,500 to 10,000 lux, and its benefit for winter blues, PMS distress, menopausal tension, eating disorders, and clinical depression is well documented by research. Twenty years ago, the National Institute of Mental Health acknowledged the benefits of light therapy. But today, many still don't realize that it is an effective treatment. If you're contemplating light therapy, get expert advice from a trained professional. The time of day and length of exposure are crucial to the success of using a light box. I've had a number of clients who have tried light boxes for energy and mood enhancement and concluded that they didn't work. As it turned out, the light boxes worked beautifully, they just weren't using them properly.

The benefits of light exposure go beyond mental health to physical health. A recent study found that women who live in sunnier climates or spend a great deal of time outdoors have a lower risk of breast cancer. Other studies have shown that sunlight helps to regulate ovulation and the menstrual cycle, and ongoing research continues to support the benefit of sunlight on bone health.

Sunlight is our number-one source of vitamin D, and vitamin D is necessary for our bodies to absorb calcium and deposit it in our bones. Fifty percent of us are deficient in vitamin D because we're not getting enough sun and/or drinking enough vitamin D–fortified milk. And even if we do get out in the sun every day, we're covering our bodies with sunscreen, sun hat, and sunglasses because we're justifiably concerned about skin cancer and premature aging.

How can you get your vitamin D and solar energy without getting wrinkles and skin cancer? Sunscreen probably isn't the answer. Some studies have found that it blocks the absorption of vitamin D through the skin. Fortunately, all you need is about ten minutes of sun exposure to get your daily dose of vitamin D, and this amount of time won't do any damage to your skin. So for the first ten minutes, go au natural, sunscreen-free. Then apply sunscreen generously.

In addition to going sunscreen-free for ten minutes, you may also want to go shower-free for a couple of days. Vitamin D is stored in the skin cells before it's absorbed by the body, so if, like most Americans, you shower once or twice a day, most of the vitamin D is going down the drain with sloughed-off skin cells. Studies have analyzed the vitamin D status of those bathing once a day, once every other day, once a week, and once a month. You guessed it! Those who bathe the least have the most vitamin D and the strongest bones.

Less developed countries consume less calcium than we do, but have a lower risk of osteoporosis. They have a better vitamin D status because they get more sun, and they don't have the luxury of unlimited running water, loofah sponges, and body scrubs. Do your bones a favor: *Get ten minutes of solar energy and put on some extra deodorant instead of showering today.*

AIRING OUT YOUR FATIGUE

If you can't catch your breath, you can't capture your energy. Breathing in sufficient oxygen is necessary for producing ATP energy molecules. I'm sure you've felt the fatiguing effects of oxygen deprivation: When you're flying thirty thousand feet above the ground in low cabin pressure, you get sleepy. When you're skiing or hiking in high mountainous altitudes, your breathing is labored because the air is thinner and your muscles are weak from lack of energy. Then, some of us have chronic bronchitis, emphysema, or asthma, all of which decrease lung capacity and oxygen supply to our cells.

Even without planes, mountains, and chronic breathing problems, we're still depriving ourselves of oxygen every day because we are not taking full, deep belly breaths. We are a nation of shallow chest breathers, never fully exhaling to empty our lungs and never fully inhaling to fill our lungs with oxygen. *If we don't breathe right, we can't fight fatigue.*

How did we become such shallow breathers? When we're angry, anxious, or stressed, we clench our stomach muscles and our diaphragm can't relax enough to take deep belly breaths. When we're concerned about our appearance, we suck in our stomachs to look thinner and wear clothing that's too tight. One study found that by loosening our belts a notch or two, we could increase our oxygen intake by 30 percent. No wonder I always feel more energized when I wear sweatpants. They're a part of my writing uniform, and I'm wearing them right now.

Let's check the depth of your breath with a different kind of Breathalyzer test. Place one hand on your chest and the other on your stomach. Breathe normally for a few minutes and note which hand moves the most with each inhale. If it's the hand on your belly, you passed the Breathalyzer test with flying colors and can continue to practice responsible breathing. If it's the hand on your chest, you're not taking in enough air with each breath and therefore not getting enough oxygen to your cells to make ATP. You have much energy to gain by changing the way you breathe. You could take a breathing class for 250 dollars, or you could train yourself to become a belly breather instead of a chest breather by:

- **Taking some time each day to concentrate on your breathing**—while you're waiting at a traffic light or watching television, focus on breathing slow and deep instead of fast and shallow.

- **Making it a goal to breathe ten to fourteen times a minute**—typically, we breathe about twenty times a minute.

- **Watching infants breathe and mimicking their behavior**—their whole body takes in air, not just their lungs. Infants need all the oxygen they can get to sustain their rapid growth rate.

- **Learning biofeedback**—where slowing down your breathing also slows down your heart rate and blood pressure.

- **Trying yoga**—the breathing techniques you'll learn are just as important as the body movements.

- **Exercising**—when you move your body, your breathing is automatically adjusted to take in additional oxygen. The more fit you are, the greater your lung capacity, and the more oxygen you'll breathe in whether you're exercising or not. When you're out of shape, walking up a flight of stairs can leave you huffing and puffing for air.

After a few weeks of concentrating on your breathing, you'll automatically start taking full, deep belly breaths—and may find that this new way of breathing not only alleviates fatigue but also mitigates migraines, high blood pressure, sleep problems, panic attacks, stress, PMS, and menopause. One study found that deep breathing reduced menopausal hot flashes by as much as 50 percent!

As more and more information is being made public on the benefits of proper breathing and maximum oxygen intake, more and more products are being formulated to include O_2. Drinks, pills, and beauty aids have added oxygen to "fight fatigue, enhance endurance, boost metabolism, ease stress, cure disease, or prevent wrinkles." A number of oxygen bars have even opened up around the globe where you can pull up a seat at the bar and pay twenty dollars for a shot of pure gas. Are these oxygen products full of hot air? It appears so. According to the American Lung Association, breathing plain old air is all we need. Once our blood is saturated with oxygen, more gives no additional benefits.

So simply keep breathing, but breathe slowly, deeply, and from your belly—and your 25,000 breaths a day will sufficiently air out your fatigue.

THE POWER OF THE PALETTE

While you're breathing in energy, look at the multitude of colors around you. Each has a different electromagnetic wavelength that can affect the visual center in your brain and activate your senses. The first color research was conducted in the 1950s at the University of Alberta in Edmonton, Canada, where it was discovered that color had a predictable and measurable affect on blood pressure, heart rate, and the nervous system. Current research at Johns Hopkins University and elsewhere has more specifically discovered that:

- **Red** increases adrenaline, blood pressure, metabolic rate, and energy.
- **Yellow** increases optimism and excitement as well as stimulates appetite.
- **Orange** activates the creative center in your brain.

- **Blue** reduces heart rate, blood pressure, and body tension.
- **Green** decreases adrenaline and stress.
- **Purple** relaxes the muscles.
- **Black** is depressing to many.

What's your favorite color? It may or may not be a reflection of your personality. Black is the number-one color choice for women's clothing. It's the "universal color" we say, but we really choose it for its perceived slimming qualities. Go open your closet and view your color choices. Do you see any red, yellow, or orange apparel? Any blues, greens, and purples? Or are there mostly blacks, grays, and browns? Have you noticed a difference in how you feel when you wear a bright red suit, a yellow sundress, an orange top, a purple sweater, blue slacks, or a green blouse?

When you're feeling low, the color experts recommend wearing colors that excite. When you're feeling stressed, wear colors that relax. The relatively new term for these mood-altering suggestions is "color therapy." Although not recognized as a proven treatment by the American Psychology Association, there is some research to back up what color therapists claim.

color	symbol	effect
red	strength, enthusiasm	counteracts fatigue and fear
yellow	joy, enthusiasm	counteracts depression
orange	wisdom, clarity	stimulates creativity, boosts mood
green	love, harmony, nature	relieves tension, relaxes muscles
blue	peace, relaxation	creates calmness
purple	intuition, imagination	clears the mind, overcomes anxiety

Don't just drape yourself with color, but surround yourself with the appropriate hues and shades of nature: purple flowers, green trees, the orange sunset, the turquoise ocean, the blue sky, and the yellow sun. Paint your walls the primary colors of nature and choose artwork, tile, and upholstery that complement and balance your personality.

Perhaps we've known how color affects us for years, well before research confirmed our instincts. For example, was a red stop sign chosen to awaken our reflexes to stop? A green light to encourage us to start going again slowly and calmly? A yellow-painted fast food restaurant (the golden arches!) to stimulate appetite? A blue bedspread to relax us for sleep? Blue is the number-one bedroom color choice. Whether it's coincidence or unconscious color therapy, studies have shown that nine times out of ten, we'll choose room colors that give us the ambience and mood we're looking for.

THE NOSE KNOWS: SWELL SMELLS

You walk by a lilac bush in full bloom and smile because of its sweet fragrance. You step outside after a rain shower and smell the clean freshness of the ozone. You enter the kitchen and take in the aroma of freshly baked bread. Scents can relax and rejuvenate by stimulating the olfactory nerve in your brain. From chapter 3, you know how the smell of food not only enhances your eating experience but also releases energizing chemicals in the brain. The same is true with the smells of nature; they enhance your life experience and enliven your brain.

In fact, smell affects the brain more quickly than any of the other senses. Note how quickly smelling salts produce wakefulness, onions cause tears, and the smell of a skunk triggers an automatic reflex to plug up your nose. Some of the effect of smell has to do with memory and childhood experiences: The smell of newly cut grass may make you think of home, or the aroma of vanilla may give you a reassuring reminder of your mother, or the scent of VapoRub may make you reminisce about your grandmother, or the scent of farm animals may bring back memories of midwestern farm life. But in addition to triggering past memories, smells also cause a physiological response that current research is just starting to uncover:

- When people are exposed to peppermint before an exam, they make fewer mistakes and have a quicker reaction time. Peppermint has been found to open the bronchial tubes in the lungs and increase oxygen uptake.

- The scents of lemon and mint in office buildings have been associated with increased efficiency and productivity.

- Lavender has been found to stimulate alpha wave activity in the brain and induce sleepiness.

- Jasmine has been found to increase beta wave activity in the brain and produce alertness.

What smells do you find scentsational? Rose? Rosemary? Pine? Tangerine? Chamomile? There are five categories of scents found in nature: floral, spicy, woody, citrus, and herbaceous. You can seek out your favorite scent by following your nose to the beach, the garden, or the forest. Or you can buy them in candles, lotions, air fresheners, and essential oils. These powerful oils are extracted from parts of plants—flowers, fruits, leaves, and stems. You can place a drop on your temple or a few drops in your bath for the immediate effect of aromatherapy.

As you can see, "therapy" has moved far beyond Freud and Jung. We now have aromatherapy, color therapy, light therapy, and oxygen therapy—put them all together and you have *nature's therapy*. And this all-encompassing therapy has a new name, ecotherapy. Those skilled in it call themselves ecotherapists, and their goal is to help people connect with nature, be mindful of the environment, and surround themselves with the forces of natural energy.

IF YOU CAN'T GO TO NATURE, BRING NATURE TO YOU

What if you live in a large city where your sight is mostly concrete, your smell is mostly exhaust, your hearing is mostly of car horns and sirens, and the air is mostly polluted? You can do what many city dwellers do and head for the parks during lunch hour and the country on weekends. You can also invite the colors, scents, sounds, and sights of nature into your home and office.

- Place artwork and posters of landscapes on your walls—the number-one request from astronauts for future space missions was for pictures of trees.

- Choose raw materials such as wood, stone, and slate to decorate your home.

- Line your closet with cedar, place driftwood on your doorstep, or display seashells on your bookcase.

- Place a wind chime outside your window.

- Listen to tapes of the ocean while you're working at your computer.

- Buy a bird and let its chirps keep you company.

- Decorate every room with plants; they take in carbon dioxide, give off oxygen, and help to control the indoor humidity.

- Get fresh flowers every week for your office desk and kitchen table.

- Plant an herb garden on your windowsill.

- Create a room with a view—identify the window with the most pleasing view and orient your furniture to take advantage of it, or plant a flower box outside a window and place your desk under it.

Any outdoor scenery can be a window to your soul's energy. And research is finding that "a room with a view" can have significant healing powers. One study found that postsurgical patients with hospital rooms overlooking a park had shorter stays and needed less pain medication than those with rooms facing a parking lot. As a result of dozens of research studies, many new hospitals and long-term care facilities are now being designed to tap into the healing qualities of nature. Some have lobbies where you think you've walked into an exclusive hotel, with exotic flower arrangements and beautiful artwork. Others have courtyards or patios off each patient's room. And those older stark, sterile health facilities are being renovated with skylights, murals, atriums, and colorful wallpaper.

Whether it's your hospital room, hotel room, bedroom, family room, or dining room, make the most of windows, views, and natural scenery. To borrow from the comedian Flip Wilson, what you see is what you get. If what you see out your window is only brick, mortar, concrete, garbage cans, and fire escapes, it's doubtful you'll feel any boost from nature. So make the most of what you have with colorful curtains, stained-glass accents, and windowsill decorations. If, instead, your window frames trees, bushes, flowers, birds, or skylines, a moment's glance will undoubtedly restore your energy and revive your mood.

It's not just what you see out your window every day, but what you seek to set your eyes on in the future. Do you desire to go to the desert and view its infinite plains? Or the ocean to look out as far as the horizon? Or the canyons to see into the depths of the earth? Or the mountains to gaze upward to their highest peaks? These breathtaking sights are provided by Mother Nature and preserved by our country's national parks. They are, basically, free, and they contain all of nature's energy.

As John Muir wrote of Yosemite National Park, "Climb the mountains and get their good tidings. Nature's peace will flow into you as sunshine flows into trees. The winds will blow their own freshness into you, and the storms their energy, while cares will drop away from you like the leaves of autumn."

He must have been fully energized by nature when he wrote those enticing words. Incidentally, I was energized by the power of the northern California coast when I wrote this entire chapter. Can you tell? I hope that you felt as peaceful, inspired, and rejuvenated reading these pages as I felt while writing them. Nature has the remarkable ability to add positive energy to *everything* we do. So go ahead, open your door to the great outdoors and let it energize *you*.

HOW WILL YOU BEGIN SURROUNDING YOURSELF WITH NATURAL ENERGY?

The great outdoors is the greatest energy source! With the following list, check all you'll do to take advantage of the powerful energy that nature has to offer—and follow through as often as you can.

_____ I will step outside first thing in the morning to wake up to sunshine and fresh air.

_____ I will sit near a window whenever I can.

_____ I will investigate light therapy and get expert advice from a trained professional.

_____ I will get ten minutes of midday sun exposure for my daily dose of vitamin D.

_____ I will take full, deep belly breaths to oxygenate my body.

_____ I will take advantage of the energizing effects of color, especially red, yellow, and orange.

_____ I will take advantage of the relaxing effects of colors, especially blue, green, and purple.

_____ I will use aromatherapy to stimulate my olfactory nerve and boost my energy.

_____ I will bring nature to me with plants, flowers, gardens, and wind chimes.

_____ I will create "a room with a view" by orienting furniture so that I face the most pleasant scenery.

_____ I will listen to soothing tapes of the ocean, rain, and other sounds of nature.

_____ I will plan vacations to the beach, mountains, and desert to take in the wonder of nature and restore my energy.

Chapter Seven

SLEEP: RECHARGE YOUR BATTERY WITH RESTORATIVE ENERGY

Cells divide at a rapid pace, hormones are released, enzymes are manufactured, the immune system is strengthened, white blood cells are formed, red blood cells are oxygenated, calcium is deposited in bones, muscle tissue is repaired, ATP molecules are synthesized and stored, brain chemicals are replenished, nerve cells fire off impulses, long-term memory is activated, hair grows, skin cells are renewed, and physical and emotional health are restored.

This isn't a description of the growth of a developing fetus, the recovery process after brain surgery, the technology of cloning, or the big bang theory. This is what happens each and every night during the miracle of sleep. When you close your eyes and enter dreamland, your body is programmed to restore, replenish, repair, renew, and recharge itself for the next day. And when you open your eyes to a new morning, your body and brain are refreshed, revitalized, and ready to take on a new day. This life-enhancing, energy-producing process occurs unconsciously, predictably, and unfailingly every night—as long as you get enough sleep to get the job done.

Did you get enough sleep last night? This is not a question that people have to ponder for long. How you feel, think, and act right now is a reflection of how you slept last night. If you're feeling connected, productive, efficient, energetic, and healthy, then most likely last night's sleep was a positive, satisfying experience. If, instead, you're feeling lethargic, muddled, slow, tired, irritable, and unproductive, then chances are last night's slumber was insufficient for your body's needs. The average woman requires at least eight hours of sound, uninterrupted sleep to adequately prepare for the next sixteen hours of wakefulness. Some need only six hours and others need ten or more, but without your personal sleep time, the restorative power of slumber is lost, your body can't fully recharge itself, you wake up on the wrong side of the bed, and nothing seems to go right for the rest of the day.

According to nationwide polls, about half of us didn't get the sleep we needed last night. Not necessarily because of insomnia or any other physical limitation to sleep, but because of the overwhelming, stress-inducing list of obligations and responsibilities that kept us up well past our bedtime. Most of us choose to sacrifice sleep to finish the report, do the laundry, pay the bills, wash the floors, or write out the grocery list. We choose getting things done over getting adequate sleep. Now, you may argue that the hours between 10 P.M. and midnight are your only opportunity to get things done without the interruption of children, phones, faxes, or pagers. Once you cook dinner, feed the family, get the kids to bed, and catch up with your spouse, your only option is to fight slumber or you'll fall too far behind in your to-do list.

The problem is that we're falling too far behind in our sleep—and it's taking its toll on our health, happiness, and vitality. Over the last century, our average sleep time has gradually declined from ten to seven hours per night. Before the invention of electricity, we lived in harmony with nature's sleep/wake cycle, rising to the rooster's crow and retiring when the sun set. Now we live by the alarm clock, traffic reports, long work schedules, halogen lightbulbs, and late-night TV. And we're not living well in our chronic sleep-deprived state. We're too distracted to pay attention at work, too impatient to communicate with our families, too exhausted to have sex with our spouses, too tired to go out to dinner with our friends, and too frazzled to play with our children. We're grouchy, exhausted, anxious, forgetful, accident-prone, and short-tempered—and in the long run, we're shortcutting our lives. Researchers have found that those who sleep eight or more hours a night live the longest—even after controlling for eating, exercise, and smoking habits. *Without sleep, you can't live—and without adequate sleep, you can't live well.*

"**Sleep to live**" should be our motto, but only 1 percent of doctors ask about sleeping habits in annual exams, most health classes neglect to mention the unmatched benefits of sleep, our adolescent children are forced out of deep sleep to catch the 6:30 A.M. bus, and we're unaware that sleep deprivation does a lot more damage than just make us inconveniently tired.

For some of us, of course, sleep deprivation is not a personal choice but a haunting, recurring inability to fall asleep and/or stay asleep. At least 10 percent of women over thirty-five dread going to bed, anticipating a repeat of last night's poor sleep performance that was filled with tossing, turning, and torment. Many factors can disrupt our sleep patterns and/or cause long-term insomnia: new infants, tumultuous teenagers, ongoing stress, paralyzing anxiety, chronic depression, neighborhood noise, a snoring partner, caffeine, alcohol, late-night eating, chronic dieting, PMS, menopause, medications, disease states, pain, sleep apnea, restless leg syndrome, shift work, and jet lag. I wish I had the definitive answers for those of you going from sleep specialist to sleep clinic in search of some solace for your sleepless nights—but I don't. And I won't offer you pills, potions, or unproven remedies. You've probably tried them all anyway. But what I will do is help each of you design a lifestyle that's conducive to sound, health-enhancing sleep. Without realizing it, the energizing strategies you've already focused on are at work setting you up for improved sleep—and the remaining strategies will continue to build on the quality and quantity of your sleep. From eating to drinking to laughing, *what you do during the day affects how you sleep at night.* Perhaps you've already noticed the following connections between daytime activities and nighttime peace:

1. **Food.** When you eat, what you eat, and how much you eat influence your ability to fall asleep and stay asleep. Think of your Thanksgiving meal: Immediately after the feast you feel compelled to lie down for a nap, but by bedtime the turkey and trimmings can leave you tossing and turning.

2. **Fluid.** When you drink, what you drink, and how much you drink affect the quality of your sleep. An after-dinner espresso can make you wide-eyed past midnight, a never-empty wineglass can interrupt your slumber with unwanted awakenings, and a pitcher of water before bed can cause frequent visits to the bathroom in the wee hours of the morning.

3. **Exercise.** When you exercise can either help or hinder sleep. A 4 P.M. workout forecasts a good night's sleep, while an 8 P.M. kickboxing class can kick-start your metabolism and prevent sleep.

4. **Nature.** How much fresh air and sunshine you get during the day helps determine how much sleep you'll get at night. Morning and afternoon sunlight keep your sleep/wake cycle on track, and spending time in the great outdoors leads to a great night's sleep.

5. **Intimacy.** Touch, cuddling, foreplay, and orgasms release brain serotonin, your body's sleep dust. A surge in serotonin right before bedtime enables you to fall asleep. We've already talked about serotonin with regard to food, exercise, and sunlight; but even a light caress at night can boost this important brain chemical, helping you close your eyes and say "good night."

6. **Joy.** Your emotional state can set you up for a positive or a negative sleep experience. It's a well-known fact that happy people

sleep better—and that sleep makes people happier. Studies have also shown that those with chronic depression take three times as long to fall asleep.

7. **Stress.** A stressed-out, anxious mind is too preoccupied to welcome sleep. Have you noticed that sleep is hard to come by the night before an important job interview or a big presentation? Or that getting forty winks is impossible after having a forty-minute heated argument with your spouse?

As you can see, the seven other energizing strategies are also your sleeping strategies. Eating, exercising, nature, intimacy, and pleasing emotions can all lead to more satisfying sleep. And sound sleep can certainly lead to a more satisfying day. When you're well rested, you have more energy to exercise, play, work, socialize, and live life to its fullest. So climb into bed, tuck yourself in, and read about the amazing restorative value of sleep. If you find yourself dozing off mid-chapter, I won't take it personally. Close the book, turn off the lights, and welcome slumber for a healthy, productive, vital tomorrow.

SLEEPING BEAUTIES AND STRANGE BEDFELLOWS

Shakespeare once called sleep "the chief nourisher of life's feast." We can now revise his prophetic words to "the chief nourisher of life's feast for females." Of course, both genders require sleep each night to live long and well, but when it comes to sleep, what's good for the goose is *not* good for the gander. We require more sleep than men to optimize health; on average, we need eight to eight and a half hours; they need only seven hours. And when we get the sleep we need, we receive greater physical and emotional benefit from it.

Why? Because our sleep/wake cycles and biological clocks are more precise than a man's. As our bodies prepare for slumber, we have more brain serotonin release, more melatonin secretion (a sleep-inducing hormone that responds to darkness), and a greater drop in heart rate, blood pressure, and body temperature—all necessary factors to signal bedtime and enter a night of restorative sleep. Then, while we're sleeping, we have longer sleep cycles, more deep sleep, and more REM dream sleep. Deep sleep enhances our physical health by renewing and repairing cells, and REM sleep enhances our psychological health by activating long-term memory and replenishing brain chemicals. Because of all these factors, the medical consensus is that women not only need more sleep but also get more restorative benefit when sleep is maximized—more energy, more productivity, more mental acuity, and more stable moods. Before you get too excited about our obvious mental and physical sleep advantage, it appears we are also more likely to have disruptions in our sleep cycles and to feel the ill effects of sleep deprivation on our bodies and brains.

Research has just recently confirmed what women have known all along—hormonal changes disrupt sleep patterns and increase daytime fatigue. We report three times the insomnia, three times the nightmares, and three times the awakenings that men do. Not coincidentally, these sleep difficulties begin in puberty, with the onset of our menstrual cycle, and continue through menopause, with the cessation of our periods.

- During the premenstrual and menstrual time, we may feel the sleepiest, but this is when we also have the most difficulty getting to sleep and staying asleep. As estrogen and progesterone levels decrease during PMS and blood flow, nighttime serotonin and melatonin levels are reduced.

- During pregnancy, 70 percent of us report that sleep is disrupted. The thirty-plus pounds we gain by our third trimester make it more uncomfortable to sleep, the pressure on our bladders means more trips to the bathroom, and the kicks, jabs, and punches of an active fetus can wake us up in the middle of the night.

- During the postpartum period, too many variables exist to determine the exact cause of our sleep deficit: nighttime feedings, a drop in hormones, recovery from labor, and an infant who thinks that 3 A.M. is playtime. But we do know that new moms are the most sleep-deprived group in the world, sleeping four hundred to seven hundred fewer hours during the baby's first year. You won't catch a new mother saying, "I slept like a baby last night." Anyone who boasts with those words usually doesn't have one.

- During menopause, the drop in estrogen and progesterone can cause a change in our sleep/wake cycles. Women who never had a problem sleeping suddenly can't seem to sleep more than an hour or two before being awakened by a night sweat—hot, wet, and sticking to the sheets. Studies have found that women who experience night sweats are twice as likely to report insomnia than women who don't.

If you count up the 450 periods a woman has in her lifetime, plus a pregnancy or two, and the ten-year transition to menopause, hormones can potentially disrupt our sleep cycles for half of our lives. During the other half of our lives when we should be sleeping soundly, many of us are still shortchanged on sleep from what I call "strange bedfellows." The curlers we used to wear to bed have been abandoned, but we now wear moisturizing gloves and socks, wrinkle-fighting face masks, and teeth-whitening mouthpieces. I had one client who slept with her hair wrapped in cellophane and her eyes covered with cucumber slices as her beauty regime each night. And she wondered why sleep eluded her! What paraphernalia do you bring to bed that robs you of comfort and slumber?

If it's not cucumber slices that are making sleep cumbersome, or masks, mouthpieces, and gloves that are interfering with sleep, then it's our partners—perhaps the strangest bedfellows of all. As Pat said, "It's like I'm sleeping with the enemy. He snores like a water buffalo, keeps the windows open in the dead of winter, and steals the covers so I'm left shivering all night. And at least five times a night, I'm jolted awake by a jerk." She wasn't talking about her husband but her husband's movements. The average person moves forty to sixty times a night, and men's bodies generally take up more space than ours do, making them more likely to invade our bed territory. When you consider the differences in sleeping habits and the number of hours couples spend between the sheets together—three years out of every ten—it's hard to believe Pat, or any of us, gets any sleep at all.

Then Pat read a study from England highlighting a solution for incompatible sleeping couples. The researchers found that the majority of couples had a more restful sleep when they slept apart from each other. So Pat and her husband first got twin beds, then later opted for separate rooms to solve the snoring problem. And Katharine Hepburn took it one step further when she said, "Sometimes I wonder if men and women really suit each other. Perhaps they should live next door and just visit now and then." A bit extreme, but I understand her point.

Whether it's because of husbands, hormones, or housework, the average woman is getting only seven hours of sleep a night—one to one and a half hours less than she needs. And when we cut our sleep by just an hour, we can cut our daytime functioning by a full one third: We're a third less alert, a third less productive, and have a third less energy, stamina, and vitality. Basically, we're two thirds of the women we could be. Just think how much more we could accomplish personally and professionally if we started fulfilling our female sleep needs.

DON'T LOSE SLEEP OVER IT

Are you sleep deprived? Fifty-five percent of all women and 45 percent of all men would answer yes. To discover how sleep deprived you are, take this assessment, called the Epworth Sleepiness Scale, and by using this scale, rate how likely you are to doze during the following situations.

0—would never doze
1—slight chance of dozing
2—moderate chance of dozing
3—high chance of dozing

_____ sitting and reading
_____ watching TV
_____ sitting in a public place (i.e., theater or meeting hall)
_____ as a passenger in a car for an hour
_____ lying down to rest in the afternoon
_____ sitting and talking to someone
_____ sitting quietly after lunch
_____ in a car while stopped in traffic for a few minutes
_____ **TOTAL**

If you scored 0 to 5, you can rest assured that you're getting enough rest. If you scored 6 to 10, you're moderately sleep deprived. If you scored 11 to 20, you're accumulating a heavy sleep debt. If you scored 21 to 24, go lie down. You have no right to be awake reading this chapter right now and would greatly benefit from shutting this book for some shut-eye.

What if you shut your eyes but can't fall asleep? Often, the biggest problem with sleep deprivation is that it causes more sleep deprivation. Many people think they have insomnia, but what they really have is *insomniaphobia*: The fear of not sleeping is causing the inability to fall asleep. We lie awake staring at the ceiling because we're worried that we'll be lying awake all night staring at the ceiling. It becomes a self-fulfilling prophecy.

Chances are, you've had personal experience with insomniaphobia. Ninety-five percent of us experience it at least once a month. I remember my first book tour and my very first live television appearance. I was a bit camera shy, but determined to get a good night's sleep so I'd be on my toes and in tiptop shape. As I lay in bed

I thought, Oh, no, what if I don't get to sleep right away? I have to be up by 4:30 A.M. for the morning news. What if I can't sleep?! And sure enough, two hours later, I was still wide awake. I barely got four hours of sleep that night, and the sleep I did get was filled with nightmares of roaming the studio hallways lost and frantic and then finding myself in pajamas and Mickey Mouse slippers right before I went on the air. Thankfully, my nightmares didn't come true, but something equally embarrassing happened that I'll never forget—I said the title of my book wrong! Really wrong. Phonetically, *Outsmarting the Female Fat Cell* is difficult to say, but it came out as "Outfarting the Female Fat Smell." My interviewer exploded with laughter, but I was devastated and never recovered from my blunder. My first interview was my worst interview—and I blame it on sleep deprivation.

When we're sleep deprived, our speech is impaired, our reaction time slows down, our brains become forgetful, our immune system is weakened, and our fine motor skills lack precision. In fact, hand-eye coordination after one all-nighter is equivalent to being legally intoxicated, and sleep deprivation causes an estimated one hundred thousand car accidents a year.

Sleep debt can be annoying and embarrassing at best and life-threatening at worst. And it's cumulative. Night after night, the missing hours build until you can't function any longer. Just as you can't compensate for a year of overeating with a one-day fast, you can't repay a year's worth of sleep debt with one good night's sleep. You have to make sleep a priority every night and change your sleeping habits permanently.

The most common advice given by sleep specialists is to "take it easy," "don't try too hard," and "go to bed earlier." I agree with all three of these recommendations; however, I also believe that the first step in minimizing the negative effects of sleep deprivation and maximizing the restorative power of sound sleep is to know your personal nighttime needs and your daily biological rhythms.

GET INTO YOUR RHYTHM

Imagine flexible work schedules, no designated mealtimes, and no predetermined appointment times. What time would you go to bed if you could completely plan your day? How many hours of sleep would you get? What time would you wake up? If you had to do hard physical labor, when would you do it? If you were taking an IQ test, when would you schedule it? If you could choose your own work hours, when would they be? When would you eat, rest, exercise, socialize, shop, drink water, and clean the house?

How you answer these questions uncovers your optimal biological rhythm and identifies how your internal clock ticks. You are a "diurnal" being, meaning that your body works on a day/night cycle, and all of your body processes are timed to keep you awake during the day and asleep at night—as long as everything is synchronized properly by your suprachiasmatic nucleus. Although it sounds like something Mary Poppins should be singing about, it's the home of your internal master clock and keeps you timed with a sleep/wake cycle that is best for you. No two biological clocks keep exactly the same time, but we're often categorized as "larks" if we go to bed early and wake up early or "owls" if we go to bed late and sleep in. Which bird do you most resemble in your natural rhythms? Is one better than the other in terms of health, productivity, and longevity? One study looked at larks and owls, testing the validity of Ben Franklin's axiom "Early to bed, early to rise, makes a [wo]man healthy, wealthy, and wise," and found that larks were no healthier, richer, or smarter than owls. Too bad, since I am definitely a lark. Most women are.

It appears that when we go to bed and when we wake up doesn't really matter. What matters is *knowing when we need to go to bed and how many hours of sleep we need*. When we are aware of our bodies' natural biological rhythm and harmonize our lifestyle with our bodies' master clock, we maximize the quality of our lives—mentally, physically, and emotionally. Maybe you're able to do this on vacations when you feel rested for the first time in months. Maybe you have a flexible schedule and can do it year-round. Or maybe you have no idea how your internal clock ticks and what harmony means when it comes to your lifestyle.

If you don't know your optimal daily rhythm, I suggest taking a couple of days to find out. Keep a diary to record differences in your energy level during the day and how sleep affects your productivity and alertness. Each day, record the time you went to bed, the time you woke up, and your total sleep time minus any awakenings. Then, every waking hour, rate your energy with the scale from chapter 1.

10   I'm exploding with endless, unstoppable, enthusiastic energy.

9   I could run a marathon, clean out my closet, pay the bills, and be done in time to pick up the kids from school.

8   I'm productive and efficient and can't wait to go to my aerobics class after work.

7   I'll push myself to make it through the day, but I'll crash tonight.

6   I don't think I can make it through the day; give me caffeine!

5   I'm falling farther and farther behind schedule—with no energy to catch up. Where did the time go?

4   I'm running out of gas, my battery's almost dead, and if someone asks me to do one more thing, I'm going to blow a gasket.

3   My eyes hurt, my feet are dragging, and my brain has gone off-line.

2   My life is completely out of control; I haven't had a break for months and probably won't get one until I'm six feet under.

1   I'm in a semiconscious stupor, unable to think, talk, or move.

I also recommend plotting your daily energy rhythm on a graph to give you a visual picture of your level of functioning. You may not realize how out of kilter you are until you see it in black and white. Here's Stacey's graph after getting her usual seven hours of sleep a night.

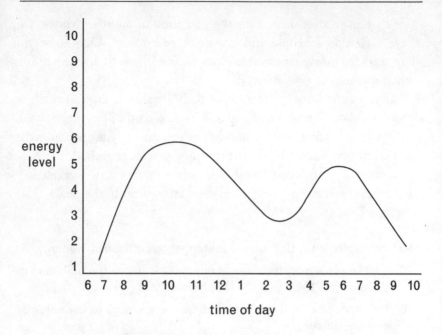

time of day

Like Stacey, most people have a peak in energy in the late morning and the early evening, and a noticeable drop in energy in the midafternoon. But Stacey's peaks barely topped 5, and in her lows she was approaching a semiconscious stupor. She was not getting the sleep she needed to maximize her sleep/wake cycle—and she felt the negative effects every single day. To synchronize her biological rhythms, she made it a goal to get more sleep. First, she started going to bed fifteen minutes earlier, then waking fifteen minutes later, until her sleep time was a more consistent eight hours a night. The effects on her daytime rhythms were evident and immediate.

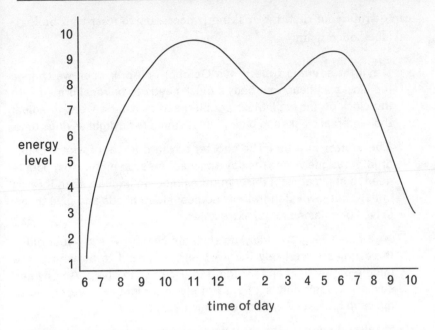

Stacey needed about eight sleeping hours to reach her peak in energy and synchronize her rhythms. How much sleep do you need? Try adding fifteen extra minutes of sleep by either going to bed earlier or waking up later and see how you feel. Keep adding fifteen-minute increments until your highs reach at least a level 7 and your lows don't dip below a level 5. This is your optimal sleep/wake cycle.

How much sleep you need really depends on how good you want to feel. As I've discussed, for most women, eight to eight and a half hours will provide adequate functioning for your body and brain. But some studies have shown that ten hours will give you state-of-the-art functioning and maximum energy, productivity, and creativity. Albert Einstein was famous for sleeping a solid ten hours each night—and he accomplished great things. Could we all be Einsteins if we got ten hours of restorative sleep? Why don't you sleep on it and get back to me with the answer.

Even if you change your sleep patterns and synchronize your rhythms for optimal sleep and daytime energy, a number of factors can disrupt your rhythms, making it necessary to reset your biological clock once again:

- **Daylight savings time.** If it's October or April, when we change the clocks an hour, your body's clock needs to be recalibrated with the clock on the wall. Most people need at least a week to adjust their internal clocks and biological rhythms to daylight savings time.

- **The winter months.** The shorter daylight hours of winter cause greater fatigue during the day and sleepiness at night. Most people need to sleep at least thirty minutes more in January than they do in July, but few listen to their bodies' sleep needs and give themselves permission to get extra sleep.

- **Aging.** As we grow older, our rhythms change. A sixty-year-old is three times more likely than a twenty-year-old to awaken in the middle of the night and struggle to get back to sleep. And by age seventy, we get only six hours of sleep a night and are forced to make up for lost sleep with daytime naps.

- **Weekend snoozeathons.** If you sleep ten hours on weekends but only six hours during the week, your internal clock is confused and you may experience the phenomenon of "Sunday night insomnia." The inability to fall asleep Sunday night is not only from the worry of what's to come Monday morning and the week ahead, but also from the fact that we're not sleepy at 10 P.M. after the extra hours of sleep on Friday and Saturday nights. Sleep experts recommend maintaining a regular sleep schedule all week long to keep your rhythms timed. This may put a damper on your social life, but it does wonders for your body.

- **Jet lag.** When you cross three or more time zones, jet lag sets in. The clock on the wall says one time, your body's internal clock says another, and it can take up to ten days to adjust to the new time zone. By that time, however, the vacation is probably over, and your clock has to be readjusted again after your trip home. Some traveling tips include setting your watch to your destination time before the plane takes off, getting an hour of natural sunlight as soon as you arrive, eating the meal that the natives are eating, and exercising that afternoon.

- **Shift work.** If your work schedule changes to the night shift, it's like crossing fourteen time zones and traveling halfway around the world. Night workers used to be found only in hospitals, police departments, and fire stations, but now they're in grocery stores, television studios, mail-order companies, Internet businesses, all-night diners, and airplanes. Of the 40 million people who work nights, 70 percent report difficulty in falling asleep and get two hours less sleep each day than they need. Although it's biologically impossible to adjust completely to a reversed sleep/wake cycle, it's best to decide on a routine and stick with it: Eat, sleep, exercise, and socialize at approximately the same times every day.

- **Excessive daytime napping.** Half of the world naps somewhere between one and four in the afternoon. Needless to say, we're a part of the other half. A short nap of ten to thirty minutes can be revitalizing, especially for those over sixty, new moms, and other sleep-deprived individuals. But a longer nap, of more than an hour, can disrupt your rhythms and hinder sleep that night.

- **Evening exercise.** Evening and late-night exercise releases stimulating hormones, increases body temperature, and can wake you up when your body's clock thinks it's getting close to bedtime. But exercising in the afternoon can help your clock keep better time. The University of Arizona found that those who walked five blocks every afternoon were 50 percent less likely to have sleep difficulties that night.

- **Night eating.** As your body is preparing for sleep, your digestive system wants to turn out the lights, too. But wait! What's this triple-decker sandwich coming my way at 11 P.M.? This is going to take hours to digest. Oh, well, I guess I'll have to stay up awhile longer.

Nighttime nibbling is not the only eating habit that keeps your stomach, and therefore you, awake. *What you eat and drink during the day affects how you sleep at night.*

EAT RIGHT, SLEEP TIGHT

As a nutritionist, it's not only my duty to educate you on the effects of eating and drinking on your biological rhythms and sleep cycles, it's also my desire to alert you to what you're eating that's robbing you of sleep and what you're not eating that could significantly enhance your sleep. Let's start with the sleep robbers first.

- **Caffeine.** Everyone knows that caffeine can keep you up, but you may not know that the stimulating effects of caffeine last longer than an hour's jolt. For up to seven hours, it keeps adrenaline, heart rate, and blood pressure high. So that 4 P.M. cup of coffee to counteract the afternoon slump may be counterproductive to sleep at 10 P.M. that night. Although some of you may claim that you're not affected by an afternoon latte or even an after-dinner cappuccino, my recommendation is to go without it and see if it helps. (Keep your morning java if it's important to you; it won't hinder sleep.) Caffeine is not only found in coffee drinks; here are a few surprising comparisons:

  - No-Doz contains as much caffeine as two cups of coffee.

  - Excedrin contains more caffeine than most soft drinks.

  - Mountain Dew has more caffeine than Coke.

  - Dr Pepper contains more caffeine than Pepsi.

  - Drip coffee contains two times more caffeine than instant coffee.

  - Tea brewed for five minutes contains 50 percent more caffeine than tea brewed for one minute.

- **Dieting.** A study published in the *American Journal of Clinical Nutrition* found that dieters took 70 percent longer to fall asleep and had 15 percent less deep sleep than non-dieters. Less food equals less sleep—and more irritability and fatigue. Our dieting insomnia is a protective mechanism from times of famine. To forage for every morsel of available food, our bodies keep us up at night to continue the search. *Stop dieting and you'll start sleeping better.*

- **Going to bed hungry.** Whether you're dieting or not, hunger pangs can wake you up like an alarm clock for a midnight trip to the kitchen. When you're extremely hungry, adrenaline is released because your body views the hunger as a state of emergency. Listen to your hunger and have a little more at dinner or a light snack thirty minutes before you hit the sack.

- **Going to bed full.** When a group of Swiss scientists fed women a large meal at either 6 P.M. and 9 P.M., the late diners initially felt sleepier because their blood supply went to their stomachs for digestion, but they also slept less soundly because they had a 20 percent higher stomach acid production all night long. Both digestion and indigestion can wake you up and keep you up.

- **Alcohol.** Even though most people find that a drink before bed helps them fall asleep faster, two hours later they are wide awake. Alcohol has been found to increase awakenings and decrease REM dream sleep.

- **Drinking too much water at night.** A full bladder alerts your brain, wakes you up with that familiar urge, and makes you crawl out of bed for some relief. On the way back to bed, you stub your toe on the dresser, cry out in pain, and can't get back to sleep.

How many of these sleep robbers are stealing your slumber? Identify them and eliminate them one at a time to note the positive effects on your sleeping patterns. Once you've deemphasized the sleep robbers, you can then start focusing on the dietary sleep enhancers. They include:

- **Carbohydrates.** A very light carbohydrate snack thirty minutes before bedtime can aid in serotonin release and help you fall asleep faster. A couple of crackers or a half cup of cereal is a small enough portion so that digestion won't keep you up, but it's large enough so that the serotonin release will put you to sleep. Any starch or fruit will release serotonin, but MIT found that English muffins and bananas made people the sleepiest at bedtime.

- **Sweets.** The phrase "sweet dreams" had to come from somewhere. More than fifty years ago, honey was discovered to aid in sleep and was touted as the world's best sleeping pill. Now we know that it doesn't have to be honey; anything sweet will do the trick. Contrary to popular belief, sugar does not make you hyper. Like starch, it releases brain serotonin and will get you "dreaming of sugar plums" faster.

- **Milk.** It doesn't necessarily have to be warm, but a glass of milk before bed may be more science than fiction. A few years ago, we thought it was the tryptophan in milk that induced sleep. Tryptophan is an amino acid that is converted to serotonin in our brains, but you'd have to drink at least a half gallon for it to have any effect. More recently, research has discovered casomorphins in milk, natural substances that cause drowsiness.

- **Calcium.** The high calcium content of milk may also be the answer to its sleep-inducing effects. Nutrition pioneer Adele Davis claimed that calcium was "as soothing as a mother, as relaxing as a sedative, and as life-saving as an oxygen tent" long before calcium was found to be a natural relaxer and sleep inducer.

- **A regular meal schedule.** Breakfast alerts your body to the fact that the day has begun, lunch reminds your body that's it's midday, and dinner signals to your body that the day is coming to an end. If we listened to our bodies' rhythms, we wouldn't skip meals, we'd eat less food as the day progresses—and we'd eat dinner at least three hours before bedtime.

Hippocrates once said, "Your foods shall be your remedies and your remedies shall be your foods." Experiment and see which food remedies work best for you. In addition to your eating habits and food choices, there are a plethora of other lifestyle changes you can make to enhance the quality and quantity of your sleep each night. Ultimately, *your lifestyle determines your sleep style*. A recent study at the Mayo Clinic found that behavioral changes in eating, exercise, relaxation, and evening rituals improved sleep without medication—and those who made sleep-enhancing lifestyle changes were still sleeping better two years later.

LET THE BEDBUGS BITE

From reading this chapter you know the benefits of a good night's sleep, how much sleep you need, and how to follow your natural rhythms even when they are disrupted. Now it's time to look at your total lifestyle for every possible way to ensure sound sleep and fully recharge your body for the next day. Instead of spending 98 million dollars nationally on over-the-counter sleep remedies and another 50 million dollars on daytime energizing aids, we need to try these natural, safe, and effective lifestyle changes for sound sleep. I'll take you chronologically from morning to night to make your sleeping experience perfectly right. Think of these as your *forty ways to get forty winks*.

Morning Advice: How You Wake Up in the Morning Influences How You Sleep at Night

1. **Don't hit the snooze button.** You'll wake up groggier than if you just get up and get moving.

2. **Better yet, don't use an alarm clock at all**. When you wake up on your own, you'll automatically open your eyes at the end of a sleep cycle and feel fully awake. If the alarm jolts you out of deep sleep, you're in the middle of a sleep cycle and it may take you hours to completely wake up.

3. **Get early morning sunlight**. It resets your biological clock for the whole day.

4. **Wake up with peppermint.** As you know from the last chapter, peppermint opens up your bronchial tubes and stimulates the beta waves in your brain, making you feel alert and awake. Try

peppermint-scented body gels, shampoos, and lotions; there's even an alarm clock, aptly named an Aromalarm, available that mists peppermint.

5. **Wake up and smell the coffee.** Just the smell of coffee is a pleasant morning greeting, and drinking the "cup of ambition" as it's called may be just what the body ordered. Your body may order tea or juice instead, but a morning drink can help your body wake up and your brain start to think.

6. **Eat breakfast.** Even if it's a quick bowl of cereal, Carnation Instant Breakfast, or a breakfast bar, your body is awaiting food as the final signal that the day has definitely begun. If you're not hungry right when you wake up, you will be soon—so take a bagel, a muffin, or something else with you.

Daytime Preparation: Keep Your Body on Schedule All Day Long

7. **Follow a regular meal schedule**. Continue feeding your body with a midmorning snack, a hearty lunch, a midafternoon snack, and a small dinner.

8. **Exercise in the mid- to late afternoon if possible.** It will remind your body that you're still awake and functioning, and will help to cool your body temperature later on that night. Your body temperature needs to drop right before bed, and your cooling mechanism works better after an afternoon workout.

9. **Take a ten- to thirty-minute catnap if you need one.** If you're sleep deprived, your body may be telling you that it needs to nap more than it needs to exercise, work, or drink coffee.

10. **Watch the caffeine from 3 P.M. on.** Unless you are absolutely sure that it doesn't keep you up at night, don't drink caffeinated beverages from midafternoon on.

Evening Preparation: Help Your Body Call It a Day

11. Eat your dinner at least three hours before bedtime. And eat light at night to avoid labored digestion and burning indigestion.

12. Watch the alcohol after dinner. If you're troubled by nighttime awakenings, the culprit could be your nightcap.

13. Relax before you retire. Make sure that the hour preceding bedtime is as peaceful as possible; meditate, do progressive muscle relaxation, or listen to classical music to calm your mind.

14. Skip the nightly news. Especially if murder, war, and catastrophes disturb you as much as they disturb me.

15. Set your "worry time" for well before you crawl under the covers. We all have worries that need to be worked out; do it earlier, then let go of them.

16. Take a bedtime bath. Submerge yourself in bubbles an hour or so before bed. It will relax, soothe, and cool your body temperature by the time you go to bed.

17. Ask for a massage. At Yale–New Haven Hospital, patients who received a five-minute back rub reduced the need for sleep medication by 20 percent.

18. Don't use your bed for anything other than sleep. No work, no eating, no crossword puzzles. Well, okay—sex is permissible and encouraged.

19. Have sex. Catherine the Great, an eighteenth-century empress in Russia, was rumored to have eighty lovers on call for her insomnia and claimed that sex was the only sleep remedy that worked for her. Sounds a little risky to me, but monogamous sex can calm your mind, release stress, and relax your body.

Bedtime Rituals: Establish a Pampering Pre-Sleep Routine

20. Have a regular bedtime. And follow it with rare exceptions.

21. Do for yourself what you do for your children. To prepare them for a good night's sleep, we dress them in warm, fuzzy pj's;

read a bedtime story; sing a lullaby; tuck them in; and give them a kiss good night. For you it might mean brushing your teeth, washing your face, setting the alarm, reading for a few minutes in bed, and getting a good night kiss from your partner.

22. **Feel safe.** Make sure that the house is locked up and secured so that you'll feel secure in bed.

23. **Figure out your attire before you retire.** Lay out your clothes for the next day so you can let go of that worry.

24. **Give yourself permission to crawl under the covers and go to sleep.** This may be the most important bedtime ritual of all. Release any guilt about calling it a day and going to bed. There's always tomorrow to complete your to-do list, and you'll be more productive after a good night's sleep.

The Ambience of the Bedroom: Think Dark, Quiet, Cool, and Comfortable

25. **Block out the noise.** Do you live on a busy street, in a noisy neighborhood, or with a snoring partner? If so, wear earplugs or generate some white noise to block out the disruptive noise. Some of my clients use a portable fan or listen to tapes of the seashore.

26. **Make it dark.** Do you have an annoying street lamp that shines in through your window, or a partner who likes to read in bed for hours? If so, consider blackout drapes or an eyeshade. Darkness is necessary for your brain to release melatonin.

27. **Turn down the thermostat.** Your body temperature needs to drop before bedtime, and if your room's too hot, your temperature won't drop as it needs to. The ideal room temperature is between sixty and sixty-five degrees.

28. **Evaluate the condition of your mattress.** Is your mattress over ten years old? If so, it no longer offers the comfort and support you need for a good night's sleep. The goal is to make your bed the most comfortable place in the world.

29. **Think big.** Mattress size is one case where size really does count. If you sleep in a full-size bed, step up to a queen. If you sleep in a queen, indulge in a king. Feeling cramped in bed cramps your sleep style—bigger is always better!

30. **Fluff up your pillows.** Are your pillows too soft, too firm, or too old? Would you sleep better on down, feather, or foam pillows?

31. **Uncover your covers.** Some like silk, satin, flannel, or three hundred–count sateen cotton sheets; identify what you like between the sheets. The better the quality and the higher the thread count, the better you'll sleep.

When You Can't Sleep: Some Strategies for Those Sleepless Nights

32. **Don't force it.** The harder you try to sleep, the less likely you'll be to enter dreamland. One study offered people 100 dollars if they could fall asleep within five minutes. No one was 100 dollars richer.

33. **Try countertreatment.** Instead of trying to get to sleep, try to stay awake. It's like reverse psychology and works for some.

34. **Get up.** If after thirty minutes you're still wide awake, get out of bed and do something relaxing like reading or meditating.

35. **Have a light carbohydrate snack, drink a glass of milk, or add honey to herbal tea.** Or combine all three and dip your crackers in a warm glass of milk laced with honey.

36. **Go to bed with lavender.** This sleep-inducing scent has been found to work for some as well as sleeping pills.

37. **Try herbs like valerian, kava, and chamomile.** Valerian is a mild sedative, and some European studies have shown that it increases total sleep time, deep sleep, and REM sleep in 89 percent of those who take it. Even good sleepers say that "they slept better than usual" and call it "God's Valium." Chamomile and kava are also mild sedatives, suppressing the central nervous system and relaxing the muscles.

38. **Try melatonin.** Some call it a miracle, while others call it modern-day snake oil. The National Institutes of Health takes the position that studies are inconclusive, and the National Sleep Foundation says that there is no scientific data to support its use as a sleep inducer. But some people claim that it helps them, so you might be tempted to give it a try. However, melatonin is not without side effects; people have reported nightmares, headaches, mild depression, and decreased sex drive.

39. **Make a doctor's appointment.** When sleep eludes you night after night, consult your doctor. If that doesn't get you forty winks, then make an appointment with a sleep specialist. Even one appointment can help; even making the phone call can help. One study found that 75 percent were already sleeping better by the time they went to their first appointment.

40. **Get the help you need.** If the suggestions offered in this chapter don't significantly improve the quality and quantity of your sleep, give your body the attention it needs. Read up on insomnia and chronic sleep problems, participate in a sleep lab, and get screened for sleep apnea and other urgent sleep problems.

On a personal note, I have generally considered myself lucky when it comes to sleep, but after doing the research for this chapter, I now realize that luck is secondary to my sleeping habits. I've incorporated many of the lifestyle changes I've recommended to you—and I now have a lifestyle that's conducive to sleep. I have a regular bedtime that is between 9:30 and 10:00 P.M., I know that I need eight to eight and a half hours of sleep a night, I try not to drink caffeinated coffee at night, and I relax before bed with a pampering ritual. I usually don't need an alarm to wake up, I get early morning sunlight, I exercise in the afternoon, and I sleep in the most comfortable bed in the world. (I have a Duxiana bed, and if you've never lain on one, I'd highly recommend it.)

I have discovered that I follow my optimal sleep/wake cycle and biological rhythms—naturally, instinctively, and regularly. What have you discovered from this chapter? If you're tired, lethargic, and worn out, your fatigue is definitely telling you to do something to recharge your battery with the restorative power of sleep. Maybe you need to make sleep a priority and start sleeping an extra half hour every night. Maybe you need to synchronize your rhythms because you're perimenopausal or travel to Europe regularly for business. Or maybe you need a power nap instead of a power lunch today, or a smaller and earlier dinner, or a bath and a massage tonight. Even if you feel that you're a good sleeper, *why settle for good when you could feel great!*

HOW WILL YOU BEGIN RECHARGING YOUR BATTERY WITH RESTORATIVE ENERGY?

Nothing restores the body better than a good night's sleep. With the following list, check all the techniques you'll employ for sound slumber and an energized next day.

_____ I will try to get as close to eight hours of sleep a night as possible.

_____ I will discover my optimal sleep/wake cycle by recording sleeping time and rating my energy the next day.

_____ I will not have caffeine after 3 P.M.

_____ I will not go to bed hungry or full.

_____ I will watch my alcohol and water intake at night.

_____ I will have a light carbohydrate snack thirty minutes before bedtime.

_____ I will have a glass of milk before bed.

_____ I will follow a regular meal schedule, with a light dinner three hours before bedtime.

_____ I will exercise mid- to late afternoon whenever possible.

_____ I will nap for no more than thirty minutes when I need a nap.

_____ I will relax before I retire by meditating, deep breathing, taking a bath, reading, or listening to music.

_____ I will not use the bed for anything other than sleep and sex.

_____ I will have a regular bedtime and do my best to stick with it even on weekends.

_____ I will make my bedroom dark, quiet, cool, and comfortable.

_____ I will get up after thirty minutes if I can't sleep.

_____ I will go to a sleep specialist if sleep eludes me night after night.

Chapter Eight

INTIMACY: TAP INTO YOUR SENSUAL ENERGY

When some of my clients hear the word "intimacy," they automatically think of sex. Although a vital form of intimacy does happen in the bedroom, true intimacy goes far beyond intercourse, to our interconnections with friends, family members, children, coworkers, neighbors, animals—and ourselves. Intimacy is simply connecting with people on a deep, purposeful, meaningful level, and it can be achieved through talking, sharing, hugging, laughing, teasing, crying, walking on the beach, staying up late, getting in hot water together, lending a helping hand, and supporting each other during difficult times. Think Thelma and Louise, Dorothy and Toto, Lucy and Vivian, the Delaney sisters, the Smothers brothers, and George and Gracie for intimate relationships that transcend time.

In many ways, *intimacy is our ultimate energy source*—outsmarting female fatigue more than food, water, fitness, nature, and sleep.

A good friend will keep you energized for a lifetime; a loving partner will stimulate your heart (not to mention other parts of your anatomy) forever; and a loyal pet is there for you twenty-four hours a day, giving much and taking little. This strategy will help you welcome the many forms of intimacy into your life by tapping into your own and others' sensual energy. Again, when my clients hear the word "sensual," they automatically think "sexual" (do we have sex on the brain?)—but your sensual energy is all-encompassing. It's your aura, your presence, your comfort with yourself, your comfort with others, your body language, and your communication through words, facial expressions, and gestures. To release sensual energy, emit sensuality, and be sensual simply means to be "pleasing to the senses":

- **Pleasing to the eyes**. Not only in the aesthetic sense, but in how you stand, move, smile, walk, and present yourself. Do you stand straight, with confidence, or slumped over, with self-consciousness? Do you move with energy and fluidity or with effort and unsureness? Do you smile with enthusiasm or frown in despair?

- **Pleasing to the ears**. Does your voice soothe or singe? Do your words comfort or make people uncomfortable? Is your laugh contagious or does it send people running for cover?

- **Pleasing to the touch**. Do you greet people with a hug or a distant hello? Are you soft and cuddly or stiff and standoffish? Do you sit close or keep your distance?

How's your sensual energy? Are you pleasing to the senses? Do you seek out others who please your eyes, ears, and touch with their sensual energy? Most of my clients say that they feel "too fat," "too old," "too tired," or "too self-conscious" to give or receive sensual energy. They cower in crowds, sit with their arms crossed, walk with their heads down, avoid eye contact, and keep their distance from new acquaintances and old friends. Often, the biggest barrier to sensuality and intimacy is ourselves. If you don't have a close, loving, kind relationship with yourself, you can't have one with someone else. If you feel negatively about your body, have low self-confidence, and have little self-respect, then you can't get past your own insecurities and self-deprecating thoughts to release your sensual energy and capture the sensual energy from others. So first we're going to explore how you feel about your body and uncover the powerful sensual energy that's buried beneath your body dissatisfaction.

THE NAKED TRUTH ABOUT YOUR FEMALE BODY

Bear with me for a moment. I'm going to ask you to bare all. Close the drapes, lock the doors, take off your clothes, and look at yourself naked in a full-length mirror. No, you can't leave on your bra and underwear. No, you can't turn off all the lights. No, you can't keep your eyes closed. You and your mirror are going to have an intimate encounter.

What do you see? And what's your reaction to what you see?

- "I see a UFO—an unidentified fat object—and I can't believe it's me!"

- "I see a middle-aged, average body that is pretty boring to look at."

- "I see nothing I like, which is exactly what I expected to see."

- "I see drooping breasts, cellulite, stretch marks, and a pair of thighs that could sink the *Titanic*."

- "Oh my god, I see my mother! When did that happen?"

It's surprising the number of women who are unacquainted with their bodies from the neck down. Our mirrors are strategically placed for only blow-drying hair and applying makeup, then we quickly dress without a glance at our reflection. We know our faces intimately, but most of us wouldn't recognize our bodies in a lineup. When a group of women were asked to identify themselves from a series of headless bodies wearing nothing but their birthday suits, only 20 percent correctly chose their naked selves. The rest guessed wrong, choosing bodies that were bigger in size than their own!

Whether we're familiar with our anatomy or not, what's not surprising, unfortunately, are the negative comments we make about our bodies. The average woman makes eighteen critical comments each day about herself and spends one third of her waking hours ridiculing her physical self in some way—getting on the scale and obsessing about the number, getting dressed and grimacing at the way our clothes fit, taking inventory of our wrinkles, catching our reflection unexpectedly in a window and frowning, comparing ourselves to fashion models, measuring ourselves against other women, depriving our bodies of food and nourishment, agonizing over what we will and will not eat—the list goes on and on.

How much time did you spend criticizing your body today? If you looked in the mirror and marveled at what you saw, then the day probably flew by without a negative thought. But my guess is that you were more likely to cringe than smile at your reflection— and therefore you're a typical woman who is at war with her female body. Over 90 percent of us say that we dislike our bodies, with our thighs, hips, and stomachs leading the list of our most disliked body parts.

Samantha knew she definitely fell into the "dislike" category, but used stronger words to describe her body discontent. "I'm disgusted with my body. I hate it and find it totally repulsive. An hour didn't go by today without me obsessing about my body, my eating, my fat, my cottage cheese thighs, or my expanding waistline. I'd estimate at least six hours of self-torture starting with my morning shower and ending with the TV show *Ally McBeal*. Then, when I wasn't in a verbal battle with my body, others were throwing hurtful comments my way." Samantha went on to explain that her partner told her she was getting out of shape, her mother told her she was gaining weight and "letting herself go," her teenage son told her she was getting old, and her gynecologist told her she had dysmenorrhea, menorrhagia, late luteal phase dysphoric disorder, and hostile cervical mucus. (He was really telling her that she had bad cramps, heavy blood flow, PMS, and vaginal fluid that didn't support sperm.)

No wonder we feel so negatively about our bodies. We start the day with a low body image, then others push us deeper into the abyss of body dissatisfaction. But as Eleanor Roosevelt said, "No one can make you feel inferior without your consent"—so don't give your consent.

The only person who can make you feel good about yourself is *you*. And I'm not talking about losing weight, getting fit, slimming down, or shaping up. I'm talking about feeling good about yourself on the inside. It's been proved that weight loss does not improve body image—but that body acceptance leads to weight loss. The Stanford University School of Medicine found that women who were happiest with their bodies before trying to lose weight were twice as likely to shed excess pounds than those who were dissatisfied with their bodies—proving beyond a shadow of a doubt that *the best weight-loss program is a body acceptance program*.

If the results of this study haven't convinced you of the merits of body acceptance, then here are some other female facts in support of ditching the scale, giving up dieting, and disregarding the impossible thin ideal:

- Although 50 percent of us say we'd surgically remove fat from our bodies if we had the money, those who have had liposuction seldom report a significant long-term boost in self-esteem.

- Those models who provide the definition of "model thin" have as poor a body image as the average Jane.

- Over the last decade, we've lost ground in our body image. *Glamour* magazine did a huge survey on thirty thousand women in 1984 and another one in 1998—and was disappointed to find that 25 percent more women dislike their bodies now compared to then!

- Only 1 percent of us can say that we honestly love our bodies—including those who are a size six.

- And listen to this statistic—women who weigh 180 pounds are 30 percent more likely to accept their bodies than women who weigh 140 pounds. *A size 18 can have more sensuality than a size 8!*

We need to realize that weight isn't the self-esteem zapper, we are. We need to accept the fact that who we are is more important than what we weigh. We need to face the reality that there's more to life than thin thighs. Don't waste any more energy, creativity, and power trying to lose weight in order to conform to an impossible ideal. Instead, follow the lead of those with an accepting, positive body image. *Shape* magazine recently did a survey on six thousand readers and found that those with a positive body image had these six traits in common:

1. **They had many healthy, close relationships in their lives**. More on this a bit later in this chapter.

2. **They exercised**. Not for weight loss, but for strength, stamina, and stress release.

3. **They believed they were good at many things**. Not just at their job, but outside their career—in their community and in their home.

4. **They focused on satisfying themselves instead of seeking approval from others**. They were their own biggest source of self-esteem and self-nurturing.

5. **They had interests and hobbies beyond work and relationships**. And spent time exploring and developing them.

6. **They considered spirituality a sign of strength**. And they got it through meditation, religion, and nature.

Please take note: They didn't weigh 120 pounds, they didn't wear a size 6, they weren't a 36-24-36 Barbie doll, and they didn't diet. It wasn't their full lips, large breasts, small waists, long legs, slender hips, big eyes, or luxurious hair that made them feel good about themselves. It was their inner qualities, their connection to others, and their sense of self that gave them lasting sensual energy. So let's look at each of these traits to expand your concept of body image beyond size, weight, and appearance—to feeling good about who you are, what your body and mind can do, and how you express yourself.

Who Are You?

"I'm a mother, wife, daughter, bookstore manager, housekeeper, house budgeter, and short-order cook." When posed this question, Chris defined herself by the roles she played in life in relation to other people—not by who she was as a separate, individual person. Her identity was shaped by others, not by her own self-concept. So I asked her to describe herself using the following adjectives, and I'd like you to do the same. Circle any or all of the words that you feel describe who *you* are:

smart	dependable	organized
strong	playful	caring
healthy	creative	witty
capable	supportive	loving
independent	flexible	spontaneous
funny	sexy	level-headed
responsible	resourceful	motivated

No negative adjectives, no negative thoughts. Positive words were listed on purpose so that you'd have no other choice but to evaluate yourself positively—and see yourself in a more accepting light. After doing this activity, Chris concluded, "Well, I guess I'm not just a fat, exhausted, out-of-shape mother, wife, and housekeeper who can't get control of her life." Actually, she was a dynamic, interesting person who found it helpful to start each day with a positive affirmation to remind herself of how special she was: "I am a strong, healthy, witty, caring, dependable, and resourceful woman—and I am proud of who I am." It didn't take long for her sensual energy to start to soar.

What Can You Do?

Not what do you do, what *can* you do? You may do the accounting every day, the cooking every evening, and the laundry every night, but what can you do with your inborn talents and skills? What could you do if you released your sensual energy and creativity?

When Chris thought about what she could do if she gave herself the time and freedom to explore her abilities, her list included:

writing poetry
painting a landscape
designing flower arrangements
throwing a great party
making the best damn cheesecake in the world
telling jokes
swimming with the butterfly stroke
playing the piano

She also realized that she hadn't painted since her twenties and hadn't sat in front of a piano keyboard in over a decade. And she missed the sense of accomplishment and personal gratification she received from doing these and other activities. To boost her self-image, she started each week by writing poetry on Monday morning and ended each week by painting on the weekend. She also pulled out her cheesecake recipe and made me one as a thank-you. Hands down, it was "the best damn cheesecake" I've ever had.

What would be on your "can-do" list? Pick one talent that's been on the back burner for too long and reintroduce it into your life. The satisfaction you'll get will add to your sensual energy. Even if you choose not to develop any of your skills right now, acknowledging them will make you feel better about who you are and what you can do.

How Do You Express Yourself?

When I posed this question to Chris, she thought it might be a trick question and responded, "With my mouth. I'm fluent in English, Spanish, French, Italian, and Russian." After adding this gifted language skill to her list of things she could do, I clarified the fact that expression not only comes from verbal communication, but also from nonverbal body language, posture, movement, and spirituality. Then I followed up by asking Chris these specific questions:

- **How do you stand? Like an exclamation mark or a comma?** "I'm definitely curved. My shoulders are stuck in the slump position, and I bet I'd be three inches taller if I held my head high." You not only gain height but also self-esteem when you stand straight and tall. Take a day and purposefully pin your shoulders back and lift your head. You'll feel your sensual energy lift along with you.

- **When you walk into a room full of people, do you feel powerful or powerless?** "As soon as I walk into a room, I scan the perimeter for thin, beautiful women, then I usually want to turn around and run out." Stay put and keep walking. Size can be an asset when entering a crowd. Many larger women have the ability to knock you over with their presence, while some thinner women often fade into the background.

- **Do you ask for what you need, or are you afraid to ask?** Chris thought about this question for a moment, then replied, "I'm not just afraid, I'm terrified to ask because I'm afraid the answer will be no. I haven't asked for a raise in over two years." Even if the answer is no, asking can raise your self-respect. And if the answer is yes, you'll wonder why you waited so long.

- **Do you speak your mind to others?** "If someone hurts me in some way, I'm more likely to clam up than speak up." Letting people know when you're upset, angry, hurt, or disappointed frees up your emotions and allows you to redirect your energy to other areas of your life.

- **Do you speak your mind to yourself?** Every time your inner voice puts you down with self-deprecating thoughts and comments like "You can't eat that" or "You're too fat to wear a bathing suit," what do you do? Chris quickly responded, "That's easy. I don't eat and I don't go swimming." A better option would be to respond strongly and forcefully with something like: "Shut the @#*& up! I can do whatever I want and wear whatever I want." That inner voice will retreat with its tail between its legs.

- **Do you belong to organizations you believe in?** "The only organization I belong to is the PTA, but I don't even go to the meetings." Passion for a worthy cause is a form of expression. It may be for the homeless, needy children, battered women, education, or the environment—but getting involved gives a spark to your life that extends beyond your immediate surroundings. A study done at Cornell University found that women who were actively involved in volunteer organizations lived longer.

- **Do you meditate, pray, or take in the awe of life and nature in some way?** "I haven't said a Hail Mary since childhood and I don't know how to meditate." You don't necessarily have to recite a church prayer or light incense and stare at a candle. Prayer and meditation come in many different forms: sitting by a river and contemplating life, staring at a sunset and getting lost in its beauty, or lying in bed and appreciating your good fortune.

- **Do you feel your body move through yoga, dance, exercise, or other concentrated movements?** "The only time I feel my body move is when I'm running up the stairs, late for a meeting. My heart's pumping so hard that I feel it pressing against my chest." There's more to movement than a pumping heart. Expressing yourself through belly dancing, tai chi, ballet, tennis, golf, mountain climbing, white-water rafting, or some other purposeful movement puts you in touch with your body by helping you feel your muscles, stretch your tendons, and command your physical power.

- **Do you make love with the lights on?** To this last question, Chris exclaimed, "Never! I undress in the bathroom, make sure the lights are off, hope he doesn't touch my thighs, then back away from the bed so he won't see my cellulite." And we call this making love?

Shape magazine reported that those women who were unhappy with their bodies were the least likely to undress in front of their partners, make love with the lights on, or make love at all, for that matter—thereby missing out on one of the most gratifying ways to express themselves and experience intimacy.

CAPTURE THE RAPTURE

I might as well get this sex section over and done with. Having been brought up Catholic, there's still that voice in the back of my head reminding me that "good girls don't talk about sex," but I'll try to keep that voice quiet for the next few pages and do my best to avoid becoming an embarrassed, tongue-tied teenager.

Most everyone would agree that sex is energizing, revitalizing, and stimulating to the mind, body, and soul. Otherwise, 100 million people around the globe wouldn't have done it today. If you're one of those people, bravo. You know exactly what I'm talking about because you've got endorphins floating around in your brain, abundant amounts of serotonin making you feel good, ATP molecules energizing your cells, and increased blood circulation making your skin glow. And that's just what happens within minutes of a satisfying lovemaking session. For days after, your immune system is boosted, your white blood cells are keeping you healthy, and your arteries are cleaning themselves out. *Good sex protects you from bad health—and may be just what the doctor ordered.*

If you're not one of those 100 million people, maybe I can persuade you to take a roll in the hay soon and add some zest to your sex life. How is your sex life? Alive and kicking or dead and buried? For Jessica, it went lifeless years ago. "We used to make love almost every day, then the new job, new baby, new house, and new responsibilities put out the flame of passion and we're lucky if we do it once a month. I used to be a sex fiend; now I call myself a sex camel—and

I'm in the longest dry spell I've ever been in. Everyone must have a better sex life than me because mine is nonexistent."

Everyone does not have a better sex life than Jessica, or you, if you have a similar situation. Recent studies have found that up to 40 percent of women ages eighteen to fifty are unsatisfied with their sex lives—either with the quantity or the quality of bedtime activities. And it's zapping our sensual energy and vitality.

If you're one of these 40 percent, the question is: **Why are you unsatisfied?** It's easy to blame our partners: that they're not romantic enough, that they don't take the time to please us, that they are uninterested in sex, or that they are too interested in sex and we're just not in the mood. Instead of looking for faults in your partner, assess what's going on with *you*. What's your contribution to an unhappy sex life? And perhaps more important, what are you going to do about it?

- **"I feel too fat and uncomfortable with my body to have fun in bed."** One out of every three women say that their love handles inhibit lovemaking. But ample hips give our partners something to grab on to (they don't call them love handles for nothing). So let them grab on tight and ask them about how they feel your body in bed. You might be pleasantly surprised. The majority of men say that they like their wives "just the way they are"—even if they are carrying extra weight. If he likes your naked body, you can learn to like it, too.

- **"I'm too old to enjoy sex anymore."** Too old, poppycock! Women over the age of fifty report better sex lives than those under the age of thirty. The worry about contraception and pregnancy is behind us, and as we grow older, we're more likely to ask for what we want in bed. Now for men, age does seem to take away desire. George Burns once said, "Trying to have sex at an advanced age is like trying to play pool with a rope." That must have been before the discovery of Viagra.

- **"I really do have a headache most nights."** Sorry. That's no reason to pass on your partner's advances and roll over, either. Sex has been found to be a great migraine treatment because it releases endorphins, natural painkillers, and takes your mind off your throbbing temples.

- **"I'm too stressed and exhausted to even think about sex."** This book should remedy that problem, giving you more energy for sex and every other important activity in your life. But in the meantime, you can always use sex as a stress-reduction technique. It reduces adrenaline, calms the body, and mends the mind.

- **"I don't have time for sex anymore."** Sex is like everything else in our lives; you have to spend time at it to make it good. Set a weekly "date" for sex, take advantage of weekends, use your imagination for new places, new positions, and new fantasies. Where there's a will, there's a way.

- **"I've lost my libido and my lubrication."** If you've lost your libido, you can find it again. Hormonal changes in menopause can cause decreased lubrication and decreased desire. Creams, jellies, and estrogen replacement can help—and so can testosterone. We naturally have some of the male hormone, testosterone, and it is a major factor in determining our sex drive. If testosterone is lacking in your body, replacing it can do wonders, putting the zest back into your sex life. Talk to your doctor about it.

- **"I'm too depressed to be interested in sex."** Clinical depression can reduce our desire for many activities, including sex. You can be screened for depression, seek counseling, and try antidepressant drug treatment if necessary. But ask about the side effects of various drugs; some antidepressants can reduce sex drive.

- **"I'm single, sick of the dating scene, and can't find a decent man anyway."** I realize that it's not easy to find someone to date or to spend the rest of your life with these days, but you have to set yourself up for the opportunity. And I'm not necessarily talking about the bar scene. Meeting the opposite sex through mutual friends, blind dates, fund-raisers, singles groups, volunteer organizations, travel groups, and adventure clubs will at least get you out to socialize and have fun. You never know where you might meet that special person.

- **"I have a fear of intimacy."** This may be the biggest barrier to a satisfying sex life. Jan realized that she kept extra weight on to keep intimacy out of her life and avoided men like the plague. As she put it, "Every time I meet a man I like, I run quicker than a cheap pair of panty hose." Do you? Or do you use every excuse to avoid the man you've been married to for the last twenty years? Your sex life won't improve until you face your fear of intimacy and overcome it.

"What about aphrodisiacs?" asked Jan. "Whether I'm stressed, depressed, or have a fear of the opposite sex, will food put me in the mood?" The FDA says no food or supplement is a proven aphrodisiac, but it's fun to talk about amorous edibles and lovin' spoonfuls—and even more fun to experiment with them. A romantic dinner can certainly be a prelude to sex, and breakfast in bed can lead to some hanky-panky. But what about the lustful powers of certain foods? Is there such a thing as Cupid's cuisine?

Oysters have the longest sex-enhancing history, dating back to the Greek gods. When Uranus cut off his genitals and threw them into the sea, Aphrodite, the goddess of beauty and love, rose from the waters, and oysters, clams, mussels, and sea slugs took on the power of igniting pleasure—presumably because these sea creatures resembled the shape of sex organs. Throughout the ages, anything resembling the genitals has at one time or another been thought to be an aphrodisiac. The phallic shape of cucumbers, bananas, and rhinoceros horns (which is where the word "horny" came from) as well as the vaginal shape of pomegranates, cantaloupe, and vanilla root are some examples of foods that were previously thought to excite.

Alcohol, of course, has been used to enhance pleasure for centuries, but as Shakespeare wrote in *Macbeth*, "It provokes the desire, but it takes away the performance." It may dissolve inhibitions, but it also decreases arousal. At one time, ginseng was combined with alcohol and labeled "the liqueur of love." And 100 years ago, cocoa was made into a beverage called the "drink of passion." The Aztec emperors were reported to drink 100 cups a day for sexual prowess.

More contemporary research on aphrodisiacs has moved the focus beyond food and drink to aromas. The Smell and Taste Research Foundation in Chicago has found that the smell of pumpkin pie and doughnuts increased penile blood flow in men, while the scent of Good & Plenty candy and cucumbers enhanced vaginal blood flow in women. So much for expensive perfumes from Paris; go to the grocery store instead. Look for randy men in the bakery department—and bring your cucumber and candy with you.

You can have fun trying oysters, bananas, chocolate, and pumpkin pie, but you have to make sex a priority in the first place. If sex is on the bottom of your to-do list, get on top of it, literally. Most women say that other activities take precedence and that they would rather be doing something other than having sex to make themselves feel good. One study asked ten thousand women from fourteen countries, "If you could do only one thing, would you choose sex with a celebrity or a shopping spree on someone else's tab?" A surprising 57 percent chose shopping. FYI—for those who did choose sex, the number-one celebrity pick was Tom Cruise in all countries but ours. We opted for Harrison Ford.

If you'd personally choose shopping over Harrison (how could you!), at least pop into Victoria's Secret while you're at the mall. Shopping and sex don't have to be mutually exclusive. Or, maybe you'd choose neither shopping nor sex to make yourself feel good. All studies have shown that our female friendships top the list of "feel good" activities, adding more vitality and satisfaction to our lives than orgasms, clothes, money, or power.

VITALITY ATTRACTS: GET BY WITH A LITTLE HELP FROM YOUR FRIENDS

Vital friends give us a shot of energy. They make us smile, feel whole, and keep us going during the most difficult times. We describe them as positive, uplifting, optimistic, and centered. We admire them for their sense of humor, distinctive laugh, sensual energy, and passion for life. We're attracted to them like moths to a light, and we want to spend time with them because they nourish our souls, put things in perspective, and give us the peace of mind that we're not losing our minds.

I often call these vital, energetic friends our *balcony people*—because they bring us up and lift our spirits no matter how down and out we feel. Who are your balcony people? They may be friends, but they can also be family members, coworkers, kids, and spouses. List ten balcony people you have in your life.

1. _____

2. _____

3. _____

4. _____

5. _____

6. _____

7. _____

8. _____

9. _____

10. _____

Now, go through your list and jot down how long it's been since you've spent quality time with them either in person or on the phone. If it's been longer than a week, you need a dose of the energy they have to offer. Pick up the phone, invite them over, set a date for a rendezvous, surprise them with a visit. Just thinking about them can raise your vitality a notch or two.

I would list my balcony people for you, but I'd probably leave someone out by mistake or on purpose—and have to deal with the repercussions. I will tell you that they include family and friends, women and men (but mostly women), and my nephews. My nephews are thirteen, ten, and seven years old; each has a different personality and each touches my heart in a special way. All I need to do is hear their voices on the phone and I'm rejuvenated, or look at a picture of them and I'm uplifted. And when I actually see them face to face (they live three thousand miles away, but I make it happen as often as I can), the feeling is akin to nirvana. If I'm in a funk that I can't seem to snap out of, my husband knows what I need. "Deb, I think it's time for another trip to Maine."

When I have my clients list their balcony people, I'm thrilled when they tell me that they need more space—their list exceeds ten. And I'm saddened when they tell me "I can't think of any" or "I could only come up with two balcony people!" Then I move on to a discussion of the detrimental effects of isolation and having too many basement people in our lives.

The opposite of balcony friends are basement friends. They bring you down, drain you of energy, have little personality, no discernible vitality, and minimal sensuality. But we still call them, meet them for lunch, have them over for dinner—and we dread every minute of it. Why do we waste time with them if they require so much effort and give us little reward? Out of obligation, their neediness, or because it's too uncomfortable for us to send the subtle or direct message that we no longer want them as friends. Do yourself a favor and focus on adding more balcony people and, therefore, more intimacy and sensuality to your life. Meet friends through friends, take a drama class, join a book group, get season tickets to the opera—balcony people are everywhere!

The more you surround yourself with positive, vital people, the more energy, better health, and longer life you'll have. Isolation can be exhausting, stressful, depressing, and sometimes even fatal. The link between isolation and death has been analyzed in dozens of research studies, and the association is so strong that many have concluded it should be on the risk-factor list along with obesity, high blood pressure, and smoking. And a landmark study at Stanford University found that intimacy lengthens lives. Women with advanced-stage breast cancer who were in a support group lived twice as long as those who received only medication.

By surrounding ourselves with vital people, we can reduce the risk of premature death from all causes by up to an estimated 500 percent! But in this high-tech, low-touch, impersonal world in which we live, isolation is becoming more and more of a problem. We change jobs, relocate, live away from our families, lose touch with friends, and don't know our neighbors. But we do know our computer keyboards and favorite websites by heart. First the answering machine prevented us from talking to people in person, then the Internet prevented us from talking at all. E-mail is not real intimacy and cyber sex is not making love. By way of the industrial revolution and the computer age, we've slowly lost the powerful energy source of intimacy—but we can quickly reconnect and get it back.

So, get by with a little help from your friends—seek them out, make new ones, and make amends with old ones to outsmart your female fatigue. Then give a little help to your friends and experience the intimacy of mutually satisfying relationships. When you offer help, you experience the "helper's high." I'm sure you've heard of the runner's high, and doing a good deed (a really good one) for someone in need also releases endorphins and gives us heightened well-being, energy, and joy. Better yet—do a good deed for yourself. Care for yourself as you would care for others. Get high from being the helper *and* the recipient at the same time. ***Because being loving and kind to yourself may be the most energizing activity of all.***

CLOSE ENCOUNTERS OF THE INTIMATE KIND

If you were to spend intimate time with yourself, what would you do? Would you curl up in a blanket by the fire and read a book? Would you meditate, contemplate, walk on the beach, take a long bath, rub lotion on your skin from head to toe, give yourself a manicure, or pamper yourself in some other way?

"I would go away for the weekend all by myself. I'd give myself permission to do absolutely nothing. I'd sleep in, take long naps, rent movies, read back issues of *Vanity Fair*, and make myself gourmet dinners." This is what Carolyn said she would do for self-satisfying intimacy. Then she followed up with "Whoops! I forgot something. I'd bring my dog, Tess, along with me, because a dog is a woman's best friend."

Our furry, four-legged friends energize us because they ask for little and give so much. They greet us with enthusiasm, kisses, and a wagging tail when we come home after a tough day. They lay their heads on our laps as we're relaxing at night. And they follow us from room to room to keep us company. If you own a pet, you most likely have a lower stress level, lower blood pressure, and a lower risk of heart disease. But you don't even have to own a pet to reap the health benefits. Petting someone else's dog for just a couple of minutes lowers adrenaline and puts your heart at ease. Instead of prescribing drugs, perhaps doctors should write out prescriptions for pets—and insurance companies should be encouraged to pay for them!

Maybe the reason we love dogs so much is because they have the life we want. They sleep, eat, nap, and play—then they eat, sleep, nap, and play some more. With an energy-sustaining life like that, if you had a tail, you'd wag it, too!

Let's get back to Carolyn. After she told me about her intimate weekend away with her dog, I asked, "What would you do if you couldn't get away this coming weekend?" "That's a no-brainer," she replied. "I'd get a massage, a facial, and a pedicure." She longed to be touched.

Do you need to be kneaded? We have 5 million touch receptors on our skin that respond immediately to stimulation. Even a light touch can send pleasing messages to our brains. And when we're touched all over, the result can be out of this world. Research at the

Touch Institute at the University of Miami and elsewhere has demonstrated that massage can quiet a crying baby, decrease pain in back injuries, increase breathing in asthmatic people, boost the immune system in AIDS patients, improve body image in anorexics, and reduce stress in everyone. No wonder we made 114 million visits to massage therapists last year!

So get touched more often—and reach out and touch someone else. Give a hug, hold a hand, rub a shoulder, offer a foot massage, snuggle up, cuddle close, and lean your head on a shoulder. If you can't physically touch someone's body, then touch their heart. You can also have an intimate encounter by complimenting a coworker, playfully teasing a child, calling an old friend, sending a note, surprising someone with a gift, smiling at someone on the street, striking up a conversation with someone on an elevator, sharing a funny story, playing a practical joke, or making someone laugh.

Joy, laughter, spontaneity, silliness—a sense of humor is a part of sensuality and intimacy and, not coincidentally, the next energizing strategy. When I first met my husband, Paul, seventeen years ago on a blind date, it was his quirky sense of humor that attracted me the most. Within the first thirty seconds of our introduction, he made me laugh by telling me I had something on my shirt and then doing the nose flip thing as I looked down. It's a centuries-old, silly joke, but he caught me off guard and laughing created an immediate level of intimacy between us. He still makes me laugh every day, and that's the real reason why he's one of my balcony people and one of my most intimate, energizing friends.

HOW WILL YOU BEGIN TAPPING INTO YOUR SENSUAL ENERGY?

Are you ready to welcome more intimacy into your life? Check all that you'll do to release your sensual energy, attract vitality, and surround yourself with close, satisfying relationships.

_____ I will become acquainted with my body from the neck down.

_____ I will value my internal qualities and realize that who I am is more important than what I weigh.

_____ I will recognize my talents and take the time to develop them.

_____ I will stand straight and with confidence.

_____ I will speak my mind to others and ask for what I want.

_____ I will belong to organizations I believe in.

_____ I will make love with the lights on.

_____ I will investigate my contribution to an unhappy sex life.

_____ I will have fun experimenting with aphrodisiacs.

_____ I will list my balcony people and make it a priority to spend more time with them.

_____ I will spend more intimate time with family and friends.

_____ I will spend more intimate time with animals.

_____ I will spend more intimate time with myself.

_____ I will get touched more often through massage, body work, facials, manicures, and pedicures.

_____ I will reach out and touch more often by smiling, laughing, joking, holding, hugging, kissing, and cuddling.

Chapter Nine

JOY: TICKLE YOUR SOUL WITH COMIC ENERGY

God created woman and she had three breasts. He asked her, "Is there anything you'd like to change?" and she replied, "Yes, could you please get rid of this middle breast?" God snapped his fingers and it was done. Holding the third breast in her hand, she asked, "What am I going to do with this useless boob?"

And God created man.

Did this joke make you laugh, smile, smirk, roll your eyes, or at least nod in understanding? It made me laugh the first time I heard it and still does every time I tell it, but that's me. Different jokes for different folks. I'm the type of person who laughs at spilled milk (as long as it's not on *my* table), giggles when someone trips (as long as they aren't hurt), and gets her kicks out of sending dirty birthday cards to shock family and friends. I think the original *Naked Gun* was one of the funniest movies ever made, I watch *Young Frankenstein* regularly, I quote Ferris Bueller often, I love Monty Python, I thoroughly enjoyed *The Full Monty*, and I was in mourning when *Seinfeld* ended its last season.

I appreciate a good joke and love a good laugh. Don't we all? A sense of humor is essential to a vital, happy life, and laughter is a basic human need—as important as our need to eat, sleep, breathe, have sex, or drink water. I've tried to fulfill a small portion of that need by integrating some humor throughout this book, but you need more than my feeble attempt at punch lines, word plays, and anecdotes. You need to welcome humor and happiness into your life every day. The problem is: Most women don't. As the trials and tribulations of stressful living get the better of us, hours go by without a smile, days end without a laugh, and weeks slip by without a happy event to energize our soul. As a result, female depression has risen 150 percent over the last two decades and, at any given moment, 50 percent of us report feeling sad. Granted, these statistics are certainly nothing to laugh about—but laughter is a part of the cure. It has an immediate and profound effect on our mood, energy level, and emotional state.

ARE YOU HAPPY?

Barbara sat across from me with a blank expression on her face when I asked this question. She, like many other women, had been spending such an immense amount of time and effort going to nutritionists and homeopaths, reading food labels and health magazines, and taking exercise classes and fat-free cooking lessons that she hadn't stopped to think about her happiness in life. Finally she answered, "Happy? No. I can't say that I am. But what's happiness got to do with my energy level, diet, and health?"

Happiness has *everything* to do with your health. A happier life, researchers are concluding, is more important for your health than losing weight, changing your diet, lowering your cholesterol level, or starting an exercise program. Happy, optimistic people have cleaner arteries, less cancer, fewer colds, a stronger immune system, more energy, and a longer life. The University of Michigan undertook one of the longest studies on happiness when they began following children in 1921. Today, most of the happy optimists are still smiling in their eighties—while most of the frowning pessimists died from heart disease or cancer years ago. And why stop in the eighth decade? When centenarians are asked their secret to a long, vital life, their number-one answer is humor—chuckling daily, laughing at themselves and stressful situations, and keeping their sense of humor.

I ask all my clients, regardless of age, about their perceived happiness in life. Many initially think it's a strange question coming from a nutritionist, but then realize it's strange that most health professionals don't ask about their emotional state. In addition to weighing us on the scale, taking our blood pressure, and giving us a colonoscopy, the medical profession should also be showing us comedy videos in the waiting room, telling us jokes to make us laugh, and screening us for depression.

An estimated 22 million women are depressed, and one in four of us will experience major depression at some point in our lifetime. Are you potentially one of them? There are many symptoms of depression, but the five telltale signs are:

1. Difficulty doing the things you've done in the past.
2. Feeling hopeless about the future.
3. Difficulty making decisions.
4. Feeling worthless.
5. No longer enjoying the things you used to.

Almost every woman I know, including myself, could look at this list at various points in her life and say, "That's me. I don't have the energy or motivation to do what I used to do, I don't enjoy what I do do, I agonize over decisions, I feel worthless, and the future doesn't look any brighter. Do I need Prozac?"

If these symptoms persist for more than two weeks and are severe enough to interfere with the quality of your life, some of you might. But brief periods of sadness, indecision, and hopelessness are normal—and just because you have all five characteristics of depression today doesn't mean you necessarily need antidepressant drug treatment or long-term psychotherapy tomorrow. What you may need is a good laugh or some other pleasure in your life to balance your emotional state and heighten your mood.

Women have always been described as the more "emotional sex," and research has finally emerged to explain why we experience emotions more profoundly than men. During times of sadness, the National Institute of Mental Health found that women's brains were eight times more active than men's—making us feel the intensity of that sadness eightfold. No wonder we experience more depression, sympathy, empathy, and tears. Research is also starting to uncover why we can be crying one minute and chuckling the next, or down in the dumps today and happy-go-lucky tomorrow. Our brain chemistry can be quickly altered by joyous events. When we laugh, smile, have fun, or add pleasure to our lives in some way, chemical messengers are released in our brain that travel to every cell in our body, communicating good feelings and alleviating depression. *When you smile, your body is smiling with you. And when you laugh, each of your cells is laughing with you—electrifying you with positive energy.*

The important point is—*our emotions are changeable.* Not with a snap of the fingers or an abracadabra, but with a conscious, deliberate, active effort. Happiness doesn't just happen; we have to make it happen. We have to seek out activities, people, places, and situations that bring smiles to our faces and joy to our lives. It could be almost anything: spending time with a fun-loving friend, playing Chutes and Ladders with your child, driving to a park, watching your favorite sitcom, or listening to a comedy tape on your way home from work.

What emotion are you feeling right now? If you're feeling a bit melancholy, how would you feel if your favorite comedian came over to your house and entertained you for the day? What would happen if you put on a pair of Groucho Marx glasses? How would you respond to a game of tickle torture with your partner? Your sadness would be replaced with happiness, your tears would dry up with laughter, and your scowl would be transformed into a smile. When your soul is touched by laughter, you can quickly go from feeling:

sad	to	happy
angry	to	content
anxious	to	calm
panicked	to	peaceful
tired	to	energetic

In fact, your body, mind, and soul may automatically lead you to laughter when you're feeling down. Haven't you ever found yourself laughing (sometimes inappropriately) at sad or stressful events? Clients have shared with me some hysterical accounts of getting the uncontrollable giggles during an IRS audit, or bursting out with laughter when they've been pulled over for speeding, or having to leave a deposition because they couldn't stop laughing. Haven't you ever gotten giddy when you're overtired? It's one of your body's natural defense mechanisms to counteract fatigue. A one-minute belly laugh can boost your metabolism more than a twenty-minute walk. Laughter increases heart rate, blood circulation, and oxygen uptake. It reduces the stress hormones and releases the stimulating brain chemicals serotonin and the endorphins. It tightens the stomach muscles but relaxes all the other muscles. Think about the last time you had a really good laugh. You probably had to sit down because your legs felt wobbly, put down what you were carrying because your arms felt weak, and cross your legs so that you wouldn't pee your pants. When it was over, you probably commented, "Oh, that felt good," and had a productive, glorious next few hours.

Instinctively, we've always sought out laughter to see the positive side of challenging situations and to make it through difficult times such as war, famine, disease, catastrophe, and death. Jesters were brought into the king's court, Shakespeare wrote his tragic comedies, and Bob Hope performed for GIs—all for the purpose of uplifting downtrodden spirits. Today, there are such efforts as Comic Relief for the homeless, Humor Your Tumor support groups for cancer patients, and laugh mobiles for hospitals. I don't know the circumstances of your life or the specifics of what may be bringing you down, but I do know that humor can help. As Red Skelton once said, "Whatever your heartache might be, laughter helps you forget about it for a while."

THESE AREN'T WRINKLES, THEY'RE LAUGH LINES

How often do you laugh during a day? As a kid, you laughed five hundred times a day. Today you're lucky if you hit a dozen brief chuckles. Somewhere along the way to adulthood, we lost our ability and/or desire to laugh. "No-laughing" zones were strictly enforced in schools, libraries, churches, restaurants, and at dinner tables. And we were repeatedly told by those serious adults:

Stop acting silly.
Wipe that smile off your face.
Control yourself and stop giggling.
I don't want to hear any more wisecracks from you.
Stop trying to be the class clown.

Now many of us have become those serious adults making the same joy-stifling comments to our children—when we should be telling our kids *and* ourselves to: Act silly, smile often, giggle contagiously, and clown around. It's never too late to have a happy childhood—so let's release our inner laughing child, heal ourselves with humor, and outsmart our female fatigue with fun.

Most women are eager to welcome more joy and laughter into their lives, but I've come across a few, like Diane, whose pessimistic attitude gets in the way. "There's nothing funny about my life. I'll never be happy, I don't want to laugh, and I try not to smile because I don't want to get wrinkles." Diane was a challenge. But even the most pessimistic scowlers have a little optimism in them that's dying to get out. She eventually did crack a smile when I commented, "There's a light at the end of everyone's tunnel, but I think yours is from an oncoming train." And she showed her full pearly whites when I told her, "Murphy's Law states that everything that can go wrong will. Murphy was an optimist, you know."

In my opinion, some of the cleverest quips are one-liners. They are easy to remember, they don't have complicated punch lines to mess up, and they are fun to share in any situation—to lighten your own mood or someone else's. I'd like to share a few of my favorites with you to see if they tickle your funny bone. They are divided up into T-shirt slogans, bumper stickers, and refrigerator magnets. And they all fall into the category of female humor. I hope you enjoy them!

T-shirt slogans that grab attention:

- Objects Under This Shirt Are Larger Than They Appear
- Next Mood Swing: Six Seconds
- PMS Really Stands for *P*urchase *M*ore *S*hoes
- **Men**opause, **Men**strual Cramps, **Men**tal Illness—Have You Noticed That All of Our Problems Begin with Men?
- Freedom of the Press Means No-Iron Clothes
- Will Work for Liposuction
- Scales Are for Fish, Not Women

Bumper stickers that tame road rage:

- A Freudian slip is when you say one thing and you mean your mother.
- Behind every successful man is a woman waiting for his job.
- I finally got my head together and my body fell apart.

- Sometimes I think I understand everything. Then I regain consciousness.

- Seen it all, done it all, can't remember most of it.

- What's the difference between ignorance and apathy? I don't know and I don't care.

- Life is an endless struggle full of frustrations and challenges, but eventually you find a hairstylist you like.

Refrigerator magnets for funny foodisms:

- If we really are what we eat, I'm fast, cheap, and easy.

- I'm out of chocolate and I have a gun.

- Eat, drink, and be merry—for tomorrow they may cancel your Visa.

- Everyone who diets gains in the end.

- I am not fat, I am calorically gifted.

- Age is important only if you're wine or cheese.

- Life is unsure, so always eat your dessert first.

- You are overweight if you are living beyond your seams.

- Diet and exercise to fight hazardous waists.

- The Joy of Not Cooking

- Exercise, eat right, and die anyway.

If these one-liners didn't quite do it for you, let's get more personal. What tickles my funny bone may leave yours numb. What type of humor turns you on? Sarcasm, satire, English humor, dark comedy, slapstick, stand-up, puns, practical jokes, tongue twisters, or tongue-in-cheek? What about whoopee cushions, magic tricks, snakes in a can, cow pie, pie in the face, tickle torture, comic strips, or Letterman's top ten list? Or how about *Saturday Night Live*, *Rowan and Martin's Laugh-In*, *Second City TV*, *Not Necessarily the News*, *Whose Line Is It Anyway?* the Three Stooges, Jerry Lewis, Jack Benny, Jonathan Winters, Lucille Ball, Carol Burnett, Woody Allen, Steve Martin, Mr. Bean, Benny Hill, Austin Powers, Tracey Ullman, Ellen Degeneres, Chris Rock, Steven Wright, Louie Anderson, Will and Grace, or Jerry, Elaine, George, and Kramer? If you're looking at this jumbled paragraph of things, people, and TV shows with a deadpan face—don't lose hope yet. Here are some more specific questions to help you find your comic relief and experience the energy that comedy has to offer.

- **What's your favorite sitcom?** One of my favorites is *Everybody Loves Raymond*, but it may not be everyone's—so discover yours. Make a point of watching it, taping it, or catching a rerun. If all the sitcoms leave you sitting stone-faced, watch the commercials instead. Some are cleverer and much funnier than the shows they fund.

- **What's your favorite comedy movie?** It may be an old classic like *Duck Soup* or a more recent hit such as *There's Something About Mary*. It may be all the Woody Allen films or none of them. It may star Mel Brooks or Albert Brooks—or it may include a comic duo like Walter Matthau and Jack Lemmon, or be a cult classic like *The Rocky Horror Picture Show*.

- **What's your favorite comic strip?** There's everything from "The Far Side" to "Dilbert" to "Cathy"—and if you find nothing funny about the funny pages and opt for news magazines instead, check out *Newsweek*'s "Perspectives" page. There are always some current events to poke fun at.

- **Who's your favorite side-splitting friend?** Stick by his or her side. Some people are natural-born comedians, and certain friends have the ability to crack us up just with the sound of their voices.

- **Who's your favorite male comedian?** Your choice may include everything from the stone-faced humor of Steven Wright to the screaming antics of Bob Goldthwait, from the uncanny impersonations of Rich Little to the off-the-wall improvisations of Robin Williams.

- **Who's your favorite female comedienne?** In a field dominated by men, some brave women (Phyllis Diller, Joan Rivers, Lily Tomlin, and Carol Burnett are just a few who come to mind) took to the stage and opened the doors for many others. Now Whoopi Goldberg is on stage with Robin Williams and Billy Crystal, Paula Poundstone is at the Improv, Sandra Bernhardt is on national tour, Rosie O'Donnell has her own talk show, and Tracey Ullman has her own HBO show.

Women are funny! And we've proved it! But we don't have to be professional comediennes to exhibit wit and humor. Here are some clever quotes from actresses, politicians, feminists, writers, and the women next door:

- "A woman without a man is like a fish without a bicycle." (Gloria Steinem)
- "I'm a marvelous housekeeper. Every time I leave a man, I keep his house." (Zsa Zsa Gabor)
- "I'm not offended by dumb blonde jokes because I know I'm not dumb—and I know I'm not blonde." (Dolly Parton)
- "You see a lot of smart guys with dumb women, but you hardly ever see a smart woman with a dumb guy." (Erica Jong)
- "I am not a glutton; I am an explorer of food." (Erma Bombeck)
- "In politics, if you want anything, ask a man. If you want anything done, ask a woman." (Margaret Thatcher)
- "When women are depressed, they either eat or go shopping. Men invade another country." (Elayne Boosler)
- "Marriage is a great institution, but I'm not ready to be institutionalized yet." (Mae West)
- "A woman is like a tea bag. You never know how strong it is until it's in hot water." (Eleanor Roosevelt)

Whether it's famous quotes, one-liners, comedy clubs, Internet jokes, or funny friends, when you find your sense of humor and welcome laughter into your life, it will brighten a gloomy day and lighten a dark mood quicker than you can say "I slit the sheets, the sheets I slit, and on the slitted sheets I sit." In fact, say this tongue twister five times fast, and I bet you'll be laughing at your faux pas, and therefore lifting your emotional state and outsmarting your fatigue.

GIRLS JUST WANNA HAVE FUN

Fun—nowadays it's a novel concept. The dictionary defines it as doing something "amusing, entertaining, enjoyable." Did you do any activity today that could be described in such a way? Or do the words "annoying, exhausting, and tedious" describe the bulk of your activities day in and day out? Is "fun" a word you would use to describe your life—or is it something you haven't experienced since you were a kid?

If you want to know how to have fun again, ask the fun experts. Or better yet, hang out with them. Kids are foolproof fun-raisers. They seem to find a way to have fun doing almost anything. They can make a game out of standing in line at the post office, entertain themselves at the grocery store, and actually look forward to winter for snowball fights, snow angels, and snowmen. Follow a child around for a day and let him or her entertain you. If you don't have children, offer to baby-sit for someone else's for a fun-filled day.

Another surefire way to have fun is to be with other women. We laugh 127 percent more than men. Let's make that 1,270 percent more! Get together, talk, laugh, and share stories. The more the merrier. Studies have shown that the bigger the group, the more fun you'll have. You're thirty times more likely to laugh in social situations than when you're alone. I have a female friend who provides great social stimulation by throwing theme parties. Her past successes include a Menopause Mascarade Party, a Stress Slumber Party, a Hormonally Challenged Halloween Party, and a PMS Parade (where PMS means "Party More Sister"). I hope she keeps me on her mailing list because I can't wait for her next ingenious theme. Rumor has it that it will be a Find Your Libido Treasure Hunt (men on Viagra are encouraged to come).

I fulfill my need for fun by going to parties, being with other women, playing with kids, going for nature walks, reading books, and just being silly sometimes. What do you do for fun? I polled about 100 women with this question and the answers ranged from outrageous practical jokes to ordinary activities that brought simple joy. Here is a sampling of their answers:

I go over to my sister's house and short-sheet her bed.

I wear my clothes inside out and see if people notice.

I wear my tap shoes to work.

I put a "Kick Me" sign on my coworkers' backs.

I start my office meeting playing charades.

I call in sick on a sunny day.

I go Rollerblading with my niece in the park.

I E-mail my friends their Monday morning jokes.

I surprise my husband with breakfast in bed.

I put cute notes in my son's lunch box.

You don't have to be a natural-born comedian to have fun, and you don't have to have a fake smile plastered on your face to be happy. You just have to become an active participant in your happiness—and integrate the fun activities that bring joy to your life.

THE PURSUIT OF HAPPINESS

I want it, you want it, the U.S. Constitution guarantees the pursuit of it—but we still have to actively pursue it. Remember: *Happiness doesn't just happen—we have to make it happen.*

What would you do right now to make yourself happy? The number-one response from women is losing weight. But, as you know from the last chapter, thin women are no happier than larger women—and in some cases, they're less happy. Happiness doesn't come from a thin body. And it doesn't come from getting a new house, a new job, a new lover, or a new face-lift. It comes from the simple pleasures in life that bring inner happiness—those that satisfy your soul, make you smile with contentment, or make you shout with joy. Those pleasures could include anything from going to the movies to going to a masseuse, buying flowers for yourself or buying them for someone else, horsing around to riding your horse, playing charades to playing practical jokes, or playing the piano to playing with your children.

Research has shown that the simpler your activities, the happier you'll be. The *Journal of Personality and Social Psychology* reported that brief, moderate, regular happiness is longer lasting than intense joy. Those with small, repeated bouts of happiness are the most content with the highest state of well-being, while those who grasp for unrealistic highs ricochet back into the doldrums. The moral of this study was: ***You can't be very happy all the time, but you can be a little happy most of the time.*** So add a little happiness to your life right now by doing something that makes you smile, giggle, or sigh with blissful contentment. And you'll be outsmarting your fatigue with fun!

How Will You Begin Tickling Your Soul with Comic Energy?

Here's your list again—the funnest and most enjoyable in the book! Check everything you'll do to bring a smile to your face and happiness to your life.

____ I will use humor to lighten a dark mood and brighten a gloomy day.

____ I will seek out laughter to see the positive side of challenging situations.

____ I will discover the type of humor that tickles my funny bone.

_____ I will identify my favorite sitcom, comedy movie, comic strip, and comedian—and seek them out often.

_____ I will act silly, giggle contagiously, and laugh often.

_____ I will spend more time with people who make me laugh.

_____ I will spend more time with the fun experts—kids.

_____ I will spend more time with groups of women and be thirty times more likely to laugh.

_____ I will play a practical joke.

_____ I will smile more often.

_____ I will make others smile and laugh more often.

_____ I will develop my sense of humor.

_____ I will add simple pleasures to my life that bring inner joy.

_____ I will realize that happiness doesn't just happen; I have to make it happen.

_____ I will actively pursue happiness each and every day.

Chapter Ten

BALANCED STRESS: CALM YOUR CHAOTIC ENERGY

You see a toddler wandering out into a busy street. You react quickly with strength and speed, scooping him up and running to the curb just in time to avoid an oncoming car. This is stress working at its best. Adrenaline and the fight-or-flight response come to your aid to deal with the life-or-death emergency. Within minutes, it's over, your body quickly recovers, and you feel good about your life-saving deed. Then on your way home, you get stuck in bumper-to-bumper traffic, forget to pick up the dry cleaning, realize you didn't call your mother-in-law on her birthday, and find an IRS audit letter in your mailbox. This is stress at its worst: the little, relentless annoyances that keep your heart racing, blood pressure pounding, and adrenaline flowing. You never fully recover from what is termed "chronic stress" because the stress never goes away. The anxiety and frustration occupy your mind and fatigue your body day after day.

No doubt, you know exactly what I'm talking about. You've not only been there, you're probably there right now, and you don't like it one bit. You snap at your kids, yell at your partner, curse at the commuters, and flash dirty looks at your assistant. Your coworkers murmur something under their breath that sounds like "witch" but you know is much worse. You can't concentrate, look like death warmed over, and feel like you're either going to explode from the mounting stress or collapse from the resulting fatigue.

It's not a good place to be—and it won't go away unless we do something to calm the negative, chaotic energy that's stressing us out. Maybe you're already feeling a bit calmer from reading the previous nine chapters. The changes you've made in your eating, exercise, water intake, breathing patterns, sleeping habits, intimacy, and joy have reduced your stress level and recharged your battery. But it's not enough. You still have to face stress head-on and make some specific changes to calm the chaos and tame the tension. In some ways, this last strategy is the most difficult because it means slowing down the frenetic pace of life and shedding some responsibilities and obligations from your to-do list—a tough feat for just about all of us. It also means reflecting on your life to separate the good stress from the bad stress.

Some stress is beneficial and necessary—it forces our bodies and minds to respond to external demands with efficiency and speed. The opening scenario of the wandering toddler is an example of when we're thankful for the stress response. We also applaud stress when we're followed by an unsavory-looking character, chased by a dangerous-looking dog, react in a near-hit car collision, or come face to face with a natural disaster. And when we're achieving a goal, rising to a challenge, or anticipating an exciting opportunity, the positive pressure increases alertness, brain activity, productivity, and ATP production—and we feel charged! Good stress propels us out of bed in the morning, sharpens our thinking, energizes our bodies, and keeps us going with enthusiasm. Think of a diamond: The only difference between it and a lump of coal is that the diamond has a little more pressure put on it.

But with too much pressure, even the strongest rock and the most resilient woman will chip, crack, and break down. The female constitution is strong, but the old adage "That which does not kill us makes us stronger" needs to be rethought. Chronic stress weakens us and may eventually kill us someday—if we don't release it and balance our lives with rest and relaxation.

ALL STRESSED OUT AND NO PLACE TO GO

In the seminars I present to women, I often ask, "Is there anyone here who feels peaceful, relaxed, and stress-free?" I get many snickers, but not one hand goes up. When I follow with, "Is there anyone here who has ever felt stressed out before?" this also elicits snickers, but all hands rise. Then my final question, "Who here feels stressed out right now?" usually keeps all hands in the air.

I guess I could be stressing out my audiences with all my questions, but I don't think so. When the typical woman is approaching a 100-hour workweek between home and career, we're stressed morning, noon, and night. We run from board meetings to PTA meetings, schedule business luncheons and home repairs, call the accountant and the pediatrician, rush to the grocery store and the computer store, clean the house and clear out our voice mail. And that's before we even begin to tackle the overflowing laundry basket, the pile of mail sitting on the counter, the thank-you notes that should have gone out a month ago, and the rest of our growing list of things to do, places to go, and people to see.

Stressed? You bet we are. The American Institute of Stress surveyed women from across the country and found that nine in ten of us aren't just stressed—we're *very* stressed. If one more stressor is added to our lives, we'll be catapulted out of the ionosphere. When Holmes and Rahe designed their famous stressful event scale in the 1960s, most women were at home, living near the support of their family, having their milk delivered to their doorstep, and dialing a few numbers from a rotary phone. Has life changed in the last forty years! Today, most women are in the workforce, juggling career and household, dealing with coworkers and kids, and punching hundreds of numbers for faxes, pagers, automated phone services, security codes, voice mails, and E-mails. Georgia Witkin, author of *The Female Stress Syndrome*, has attempted to update the stress scale for contemporary women. After polling 2,300 women, she added these stressors (among many more) to our stress toll:

commuting to work

remarrying

dealing with stepchildren

single parenting

parenting parents

raising teenagers

finding child care

finding a nursing home for our parents

finding a therapist for ourselves

infertility

car problems

sex discrimination

racial discrimination

sexually transmitted diseases

"What about men?" asked Elena. "Shouldn't they be added to our list of stressors?" That probably depends on the type of men in your life. Research has found that if you're married to a type A workaholic, you'll have a higher stress level and a higher risk of heart disease. But even if you're not married or your spouse isn't the high-strung type, men can still stress us out. The University of Michigan reported on the more general male behaviors likely to stress out women: condescension, inconsiderateness, sexual aggressiveness, and unfaithfulness. I'd like to add a fifth to this list: their ability to control the stressors in their life. The fact that they can let go of stress while I can't stresses me out.

When a group at Harvard University asked couples to keep a stress diary, men reported only a handful of stressors, while our sources of stress reached epic proportions. The conclusion of this research: Men stress out about one thing at a time—an airline flight that morning, a job interview that day, or the Superbowl that weekend. Women, on the other hand, stress out about everything and everybody all at once: their dirty house, their career path, their husband's job interview, their child's health, their sister's divorce, their parent's long-term care, their community's crime, their nation's economy, and their environment's decay. We stress out on a global level and feel the stress of the world, presumably because we have a more all-encompassing view (as opposed to a man's more narrow view) of life.

But the stress of the world is just too much for one woman to handle. It builds without any reprieve, and our physical and psychological health is compromised. There have been enough medical research, media coverage, and self-help books on the subject so that I'm sure you're familiar with the negative effects of stress on your heart, digestive system, and immune system. But you may not be familiar with some of the more recent links between stress and ill health that may be affecting you right now:

- **Stress shrinks your brain.** In particular, the part of your brain devoted to memory and learning. Brain cells die, forgetfulness sets in, and new information goes in one ear and out the other.

- **Stress thins your hair.** A constant release of stress hormones causes your hair follicles to go dormant and, eventually, your hair to start falling out. Because of stress, some experts believe that baldness may soon become a female trait—and The Hair Club for Men will have to change its name.

- **Stress makes you fat.** A constant release of stress hormones can stimulate your fat cells to store more fat. Those in your waist grow the largest because they are nearest the liver and can quickly be called upon for the next stressful situation. Can't zip your jeans? You can start blaming it on stress.

- **Stress makes you eat fat.** A Yale University study had women give a speech and then monitored their stress hormones and eating habits. The higher their hormone levels during the speech, the higher their fat intake at the reception after.

- **Stress wreaks havoc with your reproductive system.** Missed periods, heavy periods, infertility, mega-PMS, megamenopause—stress definitely hits us below the belt. It has been found to decrease estrogen levels, shorten our monthly cycles, and interfere with ovulation.

Stress causes weight gain, infertility, memory loss, and hair loss—and then the expanding waistline, difficulty conceiving, forgetfulness, and pending baldness cause even more stress. Ironically, *stress causes stress.* It's an endless cycle that will keep wearing out your body and mind—until you do something to break out of it.

LIFE IN PROGRESS, SLOW DOWN

I saw these simple words on a bumper sticker years ago, and they stuck in my mind as a wonderful life motto. Life passes us by quickly enough. And when we're under stress, the days, months, and years fly by—and we are moving too fast to remember much of it or truly experience it. As John Lennon famously said, "Life is something that happens to us while we're busy doing other things." And his early death is a reminder that life is uncertain, short, and precious.

How quickly is life passing you by? Like a slow stroll, a trot, a gallop, or a high-speed train where everything out the window is a blur? Think about your female friends. When was the last time you called one, inquiring about what she's been up to and got a response like, "Oh, I've been hanging out, relaxing, reading, gardening, and going to the movies. Hey, I'm free tonight. Want to get together for dinner?" It's laughable even to imagine, and enviable if it's true.

More likely, the response would be "I've been going a hundred miles an hour, incredibly busy with work, my son's school play, and my dad's retirement party. I'm sorry I haven't had the time to be in touch and maybe we can get together for dinner next month when my schedule's not so crazy. Oops, gotta go—there's someone at the door." Click.

Where are we all going so fast? If we were headed for Tahiti or some other stress-free destination, I could understand our hurried pace. But most of us are "busy going nowhere" and trying to do everything at warp speed. We drive fast, we get dressed fast, we shower fast, we read fast, we talk fast, we cook fast, and we eat fast. The average person takes only seven minutes to eat a meal, one third of the time recommended for adequate, healthy digestion. Then after dinner, we even brush our teeth too quickly. Although we've been repeatedly told by our dentists that it takes at least two full minutes of brushing to adequately remove plaque, the average tooth-brushing session is only forty-five seconds. Whatever we're doing, we have to hurry up and get it done quickly so we can move on to the next thing we have to do.

If we don't purposefully slow down, our bodies will make us slow down. A migraine, a broken bone, back pain, the flu, or some other ailment will force us to stay put, lie on the couch, and sleep in. I don't think it's a coincidence that stress eventually compromises our health. It's a defense mechanism to make us slow down.

Don't wait for a health problem to stop you in your tracks! Put on the emergency brake now before your body does it for you. Slow down your pace of life with these suggestions:

- **Establish your own blue laws again.** Remember how Sundays used to be? Slow, quiet, contemplative. Maybe starting with church in the morning, then dinner at Grandma's or a picnic in the park. We had no choice but to relax at home or at someone else's house. All the stores were closed because of the blue laws. Now the malls are jam-packed, the grocery stores are open twenty-four hours a day, we spend the day playing catch-up, and Sundays are no longer distinguishable from Saturdays. Maybe we could handle the fast-paced workweek better if we had at least one day of rest.

- **Envision a sign that reads "Rest area 2 hours ahead."** If you can't slow down when you need to, give yourself something on the horizon to look forward to. If you can't stop to rest right now, pick a time later in the day.

- **Count to ten.** Or 100 during extremely stressful situations. Counting is a relaxation technique that has been found to counteract the stress response.

- **Take an at-home vacation.** Vacations can be just as stressful as a workweek with the planning and preparation, not to mention the pile of mail and mounds of laundry awaiting our return. Since it takes only three days for the vacation afterglow to wear off, try staying home for a change—but still tell everyone else you're away.

- **Meditate.** It slows down your brain waves, your heart rate, and your blood pressure. Thousands are doing it right now because it works. Some women do transcendental meditation, others do focused breathing or hatha yoga. Mind/body guru Joan Borysenko's favorite form of meditation is to "eat a nice piece of chocolate cake with immense concentration."

Now that's my kind of meditation! So is sipping wine in front of a roaring fire, getting engrossed in a page-turning book, and sitting on a rock at the beach or a bench in the park. *Anything that slows you down, clears your thoughts, focuses your attention, and takes your mind off of the craziness of life is meditation.*

YOUR NOT-TO-DO LIST

Are you ready to discuss the possibility of doing less, cutting back, trimming your calendar, lightening your workload, and shedding obligations? Most women say, "Of course I'm ready, but it's impossible, forget it, I can't do less, there's no way." Please don't stress-out about reducing stress. I'm not asking you to do less right now. I'm just asking you to open yourself up to the possibility in the near future.

Some women have already entered the brave new world of doing less. They've demanded a four-day workweek, figured out a way to work at home, or quit altogether to start their own part-time business or raise their children full time. But you don't necessarily have to go to these extremes. You just have to think about setting some limits and making future changes to your life that add up to **LESS**:

- **L**et someone else do it.—Delegate some responsibilities to family members and outside help. Your seven-year-old son can start watering the plants, your husband can take over paying the bills, a cleaning service can start coming twice a month, and the neighbor can trade off with baby-sitting.

- **E**liminate unfulfilling obligations.—Resign from a committee, a board, or a project that you find tedious and unrewarding. Stop meeting for dinner once a month that friend you really don't enjoy spending time with. Change your mind about a fund-raiser you agreed to chair—it's a woman's prerogative.

- **S**chedule your calendar as you see fit.—Free up time by asking what needs to be done right now. What can wait an hour? What can wait until tomorrow? What can wait until next week? What can wait forever? Schedule in your priorities first (like exercising, reading time, facials, and massages), then tackle work and household duties. Cancel or reschedule an appointment or luncheon—your friend or coworker may be just as relieved as you are to have the extra time on her hands.

- **S**tart saying "no."—This is one of the most feared and least used words in the female vocabulary.

Are you a "yes woman"? How many times have you said "yes" when you'd rather have said "no"—and regretted it later? Hundreds? Thousands? We can hear ourselves now:

- "Yes, I'll lend you my favorite sweater [even though you still have my favorite blouse that I loaned you a year ago]."

- "Yes, I'll take over that project [even though I'm overseeing thirteen projects already]."

- "Yes, I'll accept that sales position [even though it means I'll be traveling twenty-five weeks out of the year]."

- "Yes, I'll stay late to finish the report [even though it's my daughter's birthday and I promised to take her to the movies]."

- "Yes, I'll take you to the airport [even though I have to get up at 5 A.M. and miss my yoga class]."

If you can't bring yourself to say "no" right away, then buy yourself some time. "Let me check my calendar and get back to you" usually works well. Then decide if you really want to do it and how you'll gracefully back out if you don't. Of course there are exceptions. If Oprah called me today to be a guest on her show, I wouldn't check my calendar, I'd say "yes" on the spot with no regrets.

You can also start saying "no" to yourself. "No" to negative thoughts, "no" to chores that can wait, and "no" to starting every day with a stressful to-do list. In fact, I often recommend that my clients start the morning with a not-to-do list. Since not accomplishing is a foreign concept for many women, let me give you an example of Samantha's not-to-do list:

1. I will not make the bed this morning.

2. I will not stop at the grocery store for the ninth time this week (my husband can stop on his way home tonight).

3. I will not check my voice mail after 7 P.M. tonight.

4. I will not buy my niece a birthday gift (I'll give her money instead).

5. I will not feel guilty about not doing these things.

Try making your own not-to-do list. Jot down five things you won't do tomorrow and follow through with them. It will take the edge off of a stressful day, free up some time, and give you a more leisurely approach to life.

TENSION TAMERS: STRATEGIES TO GO FROM
Stressed TO *STRESSED*

So far, we've discussed slowing down, saying no, and doing less. All of these will greatly calm your chaotic energy and help you to achieve balanced stress. But there will always be times when our lives seem out of control and stress gets the better of us. So you also need some effective coping skills to silence the stress response and tame the tension.

What's your current way to tame tension? The top three responses from women are shopping, exercise, and laughter. I think I've talked enough about exercise and laughter in the previous chapters—both are great stressbusters and I encourage you to review those pages. But let's discuss what my friends call "retail therapy." When the going gets tough, the tough go shopping. Unless you're shopping for a bathing suit (a very stressful experience for most of us), buying a little something for yourself can make you feel good and take you away from your stressors for an hour or so. But there may be more to retail therapy than the pleasure of buying a new outfit—the outfit itself may tame tension. Silky, soft fabrics have been found to slow brain waves, and calming colors like blue and green can relax the mind.

Hundreds of books have offered thousands of stress-management techniques. I encourage you to read some if you haven't already. Anything that releases negative stressful energy, combats feelings of helplessness, and helps you feel in control will serve as a tension tamer. Here are five that I tend to rely on:

1. **Beat stress with your bare hands.** Massage your forehead, neck, and shoulders to relax. Or get physical—squeeze a rubber ball, throw a Nerf ball, or punch a pillow to release tension.

2. **Shout it out.** Scream, rant, yell, rave. If your neighbors gossip, do it in your car with the windows rolled up.

3. **Make a molehill out of a mountain.** Ask yourself the question, "Is this stressful situation really going to matter a year from now?" Ninety-nine percent of the time the answer will be "no" and you'll realize that the dent in your car, the argument with your mother, or the new gray hair you found really isn't worth stressing over.

4. **Make a short story long.** Talk about your stress with a good friend. Take as much time as you need to vent, complain, and use talk therapy to make your stressful day less stressful.

5. **Use virtual vitality.** It's the next best thing to being there. Close your eyes and imagine yourself in the most peaceful place you've ever been. The stress will disappear, at least while you're there.

Sometimes the best way to cope with stress is to acknowledge and accept it, especially if circumstances can't be changed and it's going to go on for a while. Take me as an example: I have a book deadline quickly approaching, my house is undergoing major renovation, my husband changed jobs last week, and at forty I'm seven months' pregnant with our first child. That's life right now. It's going to be a bit overwhelming, chaotic, disorganized, dusty, and uncertain. And there's nothing I can do about it except do my best to calm the chaotic energy and take care of myself the best I can. When there are times in life where it seems you have no choice but to "do it all," at least make sure the "all" includes taking care of *you*.

HOW WILL YOU BEGIN CALMING YOUR CHAOTIC ENERGY?

This may be your last strategy and your last list, but the changes you make may be the most important in outsmarting your female fatigue. Check all that you will do to tame tension, silence stress, and slow down the hectic, exhausting pace of life.

_____ I will acknowledge the amount of stress in my life and realize that it won't subside until I do something about it.

_____ I will live the motto "Life in progress, slow down."

_____ I will reestablish Sunday (or any other day of the week) as a rest day.

_____ I will designate ten-minute rest periods throughout the day to de-stress and rejuvenate.

_____ I will take an at-home vacation.

_____ I will meditate to clear my thoughts and take my mind off the craziness of life.

_____ I will be open to the possibility of doing less and lightening my workload.

_____ I will ask for help and let someone else take over some household responsibilities.

_____ I will schedule my calendar as I see fit.

_____ I will start saying "no" to things I don't want to do.

_____ I will start each morning with a not-to-do list.

_____ I will beat stress with my bare hands by punching a pillow or squeezing a ball.

_____ I will make a molehill out of a mountain by asking the question "Is this stressful situation really going to matter a year from now?"

_____ I will talk to a good friend when my life seems out of control.

_____ I will use visualization to calm stress.

Chapter Eleven

MASTERING YOUR
FEMALE POWER FOR
LIFELONG VITALITY

Who can declare the record for longest-living person in the world? Who can survive the longest famine? Who can run the longest distance? Who can endure the most pain? Who can remember the most names, dates, places, and car key locations?

Women can. We have the biological makeup, emotional fortitude, and physical endurance to outlive, outrun, and outperform men in almost every situation—as long as we outsmart our fatigue, find our vitality within, and take care of ourselves for the rest of our lives.

The best example to date of our lasting vitality is Jeanne Calment, the oldest person recorded and authenticated, who died in 1997 at the age of 122. She rode her bike until she was 115, spent much time outdoors, had many friends and loved ones, laughed regularly, and ate a wide variety of fresh fruits and vegetables and whole grains. She didn't have to read a book to discover her secret to longevity. She followed her common sense and instincts with the 8 energizing strategies for lifelong vitality.

You may or may not wish to break her record, but you, too, have the common sense and knowledge to live as long and as well as you can. Along with good genes and good luck, a good lifestyle and a good attitude will allow you to reach your maximum longevity potential with health, mobility, gusto, and strength. Recent studies on twins have found that only 20 percent of how long we live is genetic. The remaining 80 percent is lifestyle and attitude. And hundreds upon hundreds of studies have proved what Jeanne Calment and others instinctively knew. Those women (and men for that matter, too!) who:

- consume a wide variety of foods

- eat a moderate amount of fat

- drink plenty of water

- move their bodies every day

- spend time in the great outdoors

- get eight or more hours of sleep a night

- socialize with family and friends

- keep their sense of humor, and

- balance the stress in their lives

live the longest with the greatest vitality and health. *Energy is life—and the 8 energizing strategies are the secret to longevity.*

Vital woman live longer because they have the attitude, lifestyle, and enthusiasm to remain active, stimulate their minds, and replenish their bodies. Who do you know that's living proof of vitality in the golden years? What older women do you admire for their joie de vivre and power to live? I think of the ninety-five-year-old woman who delivers my newspaper every day with a huge smile and a hearty hello. I also think of my aunt Gladys, who has survived the Holocaust, the death of two husbands, and breast cancer—and is still going strong. These are the types of women we admire and hope to follow as we approach our golden years.

Whether you're in your twenties, forties, or sixties, you have what it takes to reclaim your health and maximize your longevity potential. You have an opportunity right now to reshape your future and increase your life expectancy. According to numerous surveys, the vast majority of us want to reach the 100-year mark, and the chances are better than ever that we'll reach that goal. Of the centenarians alive today, we outnumber men nine to one. But as Elizabeth Somer so accurately points out in her book *Age-Proof Your Body*, living longer is not necessarily the ultimate goal; what most of us want is "to live those extra years vitally" with mobility, independence, and good health. To maximize your longevity potential and achieve your full vitality, you have to take care of your body by replenishing it today and every day from this point forth. So let's reassess your energy-balance equation and fine-tune the 8 energizing strategies so that you can reap all the benefits from outsmarting your fatigue. Not just for a vital, productive day—but for a healthy, productive life.

WHAT IS YOUR FATIGUE TRYING TO TELL YOU NOW?

How do you feel now compared to when you started this book? Motivated by the promise of lifelong vitality? Empowered by the 8 energizing strategies? Energized by the knowledge you've gained and the changes you've already made? On this familiar scale of 1 to 10, check in with your level of fatigue and rate your energy.

10 I'm exploding with endless, unstoppable, enthusiastic energy.

9 I could run a marathon, clean out my closet, pay the bills, and be done in time to pick up the kids from school.

8 I'm productive and efficient and can't wait to go to my aerobics class after work.

7 I'll push myself to make it through the day, but I'll crash tonight.

6 I don't think I can make it through the day; give me caffeine!!

5 I'm falling farther and farther behind schedule—with no energy to catch up. Where did the time go?

4 I'm running out of gas, my battery's almost dead, and if someone asks me to do one more thing, I'm going to blow a gasket.

3 My eyes hurt, my feet are dragging, and my brain has gone off-line.

2 My life is completely out of control; I haven't had a break for months and probably won't get one until I'm six feet under.

1 I'm in a semiconscious stupor, unable to think, talk, or move.

I hope you all feel that your energy level is at least a notch or two higher, and some of you may have even jumped to a level 8, but how high you go depends on how much you've implemented from the strategies thus far and how much you will change in the future. If you don't feel significantly energized yet, don't worry. You will soon. Some days are always better than others, so just take a deep breath, acknowledge your fatigue, and listen to what your body is trying to tell you to do to replenish your energy. What's most important is that you keep moving in the right direction to balance your energy equation so that the energy you give your body is at least equal to the energy you're expending.

Do you feel that your energy equation is at least slightly more balanced? Perhaps it used to look like this

energy in < ENERGY OUT

because you skipped meals, drank diet sodas, didn't exercise, stayed indoors for days, didn't laugh, seldom socialized, barely got six hours of sleep a night, and worked twelve hours a day with little or no rest. But now, as a result of reading this book, your equation hopefully looks a little more like this

ENERGY IN < ENERGY OUT

and you're starting to feel more balanced, with added stamina and less stress. And as you continue following the 8 energizing strategies, your energy equation will eventually look like this

ENERGY IN = ENERGY OUT

because you'll be consistently replenishing your body with caloric, hydraulic, physical, natural, restorative, sensual, and comic energy. *You'll have freed yourself from fatigue and found your full vitality within.*

I don't expect you to have a perfectly balanced energy equation at this point, so I hope you don't expect it for yourself. You've just begun to outsmart your female fatigue. The key is to continue making changes in the 8 energizing strategies so that your energy equation will be balanced for a long, vital, happy, and healthy life.

Back in chapter 2, you filled out some questionnaires on the 8 strategies. Without looking back, I want you to answer the questions again to assess how much your attitudes and habits have changed as a result of reading this book, and what strategies you need to focus on in the future. If you have read this book in two or three days, give yourself at least a month to make some changes in your life with the techniques you identified at the end of each of the strategy chapters. Then, when you're ready, compare the number of "yes" answers today with your initial questionnaire responses.

STRATEGY 1: FOOD
DO YOU NEED TO SINK YOUR TEETH INTO CALORIC ENERGY?

	yes	no
1. Is losing weight more important than gaining energy?	___	___
2. Do you often skip meals?	___	___
3. Is "eating enjoyment" something you haven't experienced since the Reagan administration?	___	___
4. Was your only break today at McDonald's (or other fast food establishment)?	___	___
5. Do you eat salad for lunch three or more times a week?	___	___
6. Do you feel uncomfortably full after eating lunch or dinner?	___	___
7. Do you eat the same foods day in and day out?	___	___
8. Are your cupboards and refrigerator stocked with fat-free foods?	___	___
9. Are you restricting calories to lose weight?	___	___
10. Do you rely on sugar for an afternoon boost?	___	___
Total number of "yes" answers today	___	
Total number of "yes" answers from chapter 2	___	

STRATEGY 2: WATER
DO YOU NEED TO TAKE A SIP OF HYDRAULIC ENERGY?

	yes	no
1. Is water something you keep only in your radiator?	___	___
2. Do you drink more than two cups of coffee a day?	___	___
3. Is your urine bright yellow and concentrated?	___	___
4. Do you sweat easily?	___	___
5. Do you have night sweats and/or hot flashes?	___	___
6. Do you live in a hot climate?	___	___

	yes	no
7. Are you likely to quench your thirst with soft drinks?	___	___
8. Do you drink more than one alcoholic beverage a day?	___	___
9. Do you drink less than three glasses of water a day?	___	___
10. Do you drink water only when you're thirsty?	___	___

Total number of "yes" answers today ___
Total number of "yes" answers from chapter 2 ___

STRATEGY 3: FITNESS
DO YOU NEED TO POWER YOUR BODY WITH PHYSICAL ENERGY?

	yes	no
1. When the 1980s fitness boom hit, did you hide in the nearest fallout shelter?	___	___
2. Do your legs feel like rubber after walking up a flight of stairs?	___	___
3. Would you rather diet than exercise?	___	___
4. Do you circle the parking lot in search of a close spot?	___	___
5. Would you rather have liposuction than start an exercise program?	___	___
6. Will you find any excuse not to exercise?	___	___
7. Do you belong to a gym but haven't begun to get your money's worth?	___	___
8. Do you make New Year's resolutions to start exercising but never follow through?	___	___
9. If a friend asked you to go for a walk, would you suggest going for a drink instead?	___	___
10. Does watching someone else exercising tire you out?	___	___

Total number of "yes" answers today ___
Total number of "yes" answers from chapter 2 ___

STRATEGY 4: THE GREAT OUTDOORS
DO YOU NEED TO SURROUND YOURSELF WITH NATURAL ENERGY?

	yes	no
1. Is your idea of experiencing nature watching the Discovery Channel?	___	___
2. Do you consider yourself more of an indoor type of person than an outdoor type?	___	___
3. Is your breath of fresh air from your air-conditioning?	___	___
4. Is black your favorite color?	___	___
5. Do you work in a cubicle?	___	___
6. Do you live in a large city?	___	___
7. If you were to look out your window, would you see concrete?	___	___
8. Do you stay at home on weekends playing catch-up?	___	___
9. Is your primary outdoor time between your house and your car?	___	___
10. Do you try to completely avoid the sun by covering up with sunscreen, sunglasses, and sun hat?	___	___
Total number of "yes" answers today	___	
Total number of "yes" answers from chapter 2	___	

STRATEGY 5: SLEEP
DO YOU NEED TO RECHARGE YOUR BATTERY WITH RESTORATIVE ENERGY?

	yes	no
1. Does it take longer than ten minutes for you to fall asleep?	___	___
2. Do you dread going to bed?	___	___
3. Has it been more than ten years since you've replaced your mattress?	___	___
4. Do you wake up more than once a night?	___	___

	yes	no
5. Do you go to bed worried?	____	____
6. Do you wake up anxious?	____	____
7. Is your biggest meal of the day at night?	____	____
8. Do you travel across time zones more than once a month?	____	____
9. Are you a night person?	____	____
10. Do you drink coffee or other caffeinated beverages after 3:00 P.M.?	____	____

Total number of "yes" answers today   ____

Total number of "yes" answers from chapter 2   ____

STRATEGY 6: INTIMACY
DO YOU NEED TO TAP INTO YOUR SENSUAL ENERGY?

	yes	no
1. Would you use a word like "disgusting" to describe your body?	____	____
2. Are you more concerned with having buns of steel than a heart of gold?	____	____
3. Has it been more than a week since you've gotten together with a good friend?	____	____
4. Has it been more than a day since you've talked with one of your good friends on the phone?	____	____
5. Has it been more than a week since you've had sex?	____	____
6. When you meet a new dog, are you likely to avoid contact with it?	____	____
7. Do you stand or sit with your arms crossed?	____	____
8. Do you fear bathing-suit season?	____	____
9. Are you more likely to shake a hand than hug a body?	____	____
10. Do you wake up most mornings "feeling fat"?	____	____

Total number of "yes" answers today   ____

Total number of "yes" answers from chapter 2   ____

STRATEGY 7: JOY
DO YOU NEED TO TICKLE YOUR SOUL WITH COMIC ENERGY?

	yes	no
1. If you were to look in the mirror right now, would you be scowling?	____	____
2. Has it been more than an hour since you've laughed?	____	____
3. Do you avoid smiling because of potential wrinkles?	____	____
4. Do you feel a blank as to what makes you happy?	____	____
5. Do you think it's immature to giggle?	____	____
6. Do you think reading the comics is a waste of time?	____	____
7. Do you think playgrounds are just for kids?	____	____
8. Would you describe your sense of humor as lost and never to be found?	____	____
9. Are you likely to feel sad more often than you feel happy?	____	____
10. Do worry and guilt occupy your thoughts?	____	____
Total number of "yes" answers today	____	
Total number of "yes" answers from chapter 2	____	

STRATEGY 8: BALANCED STRESS
DO YOU NEED TO CALM YOUR CHAOTIC ENERGY?

	yes	no
1. Do you believe that a woman's work is never done?	____	____
2. Do you work more than ten hours a day both in and out of the home?	____	____
3. Do you keep saying "yes" when you'd rather say "no"?	____	____
4. Has it been more than a year since you've taken a vacation, even a weekend away?	____	____
5. Are there not enough hours in the day?	____	____
6. Are you busy going nowhere?	____	____

	yes	no
7. Would you choose getting things done over getting together with a friend?	___	___
8. Is your calendar booked weeks in advance?	___	___
9. Are you either going 100 miles an hour or conked out with a dead battery?	___	___
10. Are you feeling guilty taking the time to read this book?	___	___

Total number of "yes" answers today ___

Total number of "yes" answers from chapter 2 ___

Even if you scored one less "yes" answer on these questionnaires, it means that you're paying more attention to your fatigue signals and starting to replenish your energy. I strongly recommend that you check in periodically with these questionnaires to see which strategies you need to focus on for added vitality today, tomorrow, and forever.

Remember: The key to outsmarting your fatigue is recognizing it as an important message from your body and responding to it by identifying what you need to do to energize your body, mind, and soul. Your fatigue may be telling you that you need some socializing or some solitude, some fat in your diet or some fun in your life, some sunshine or some sleep, some excitement or some exercise.

What is your fatigue trying to tell you right at this moment?

Drop everything and go do it—you'll be one step closer toward mastering your female power for lifelong vitality.

TO EACH HER OWN

We each have a different life situation, personality, change process, and health profile. Therefore, each of us will outsmart our fatigue in a different way. You may make changes right away or slowly, over time. You may use all 8 strategies or primarily 1 or 2. You may read this book in one day or keep it as a reference for the next several decades. However you use this book, make sure that you tailor it to your needs and use it to get what you want out of life.

What do you want out of life? What's on your wish list? When I ask women this question, their first response is usually a thinner body, a more youthful appearance, and more money in the bank. But on further reflection, we want more than the superficial goals of thinness, youth, and fat bank accounts—we want inner peace, good health, good friends, and a touch of happiness in our lives.

So let's rephrase the question: If you were on your deathbed (a morbid scenario, but sometimes necessary to put things in perspective), with a week to live, what would you wish for? Would you wish that you weighed fifteen pounds less, or would you wish for more quality time with family and friends? Would you wish you maintained a cleaner house, or a calmer life? Would you wish you had fewer wrinkles on your face, or more twinkle in your eyes? Would you wish you had worked harder, or played harder? Would you wish you had achieved a million dollars, or a million laughs?

Phyllis thought about these questions and responded, "I know exactly what I'd wish for. I'd wish I had worked less, had more fun, eaten more chocolate, and drunk more champagne. I'd wish I hadn't taken life so seriously and wasted so much time being stressed out. And above all, I'd wish that I had cherished every waking moment."

Don't wait until it's too late! Think about what you want out of life—and go after it now! You won't miraculously wake up to a less hectic schedule tomorrow; you have to purposefully slow down. You won't spontaneously have more energy in the next hour; you have to help your body manufacture it. You can't snap your fingers and feel more content with life; you have to add happiness to each day. You have the knowledge, you have the tools, and you have a vitality-enhancing plan with the 8 energizing strategies. Now it's up to you to grasp the natural energy sources, balance your energy equation, and achieve lifelong vitality. It's up to you to actively pursue life and shape it as you see fit.

8 natural → energy equation → fatigue → lifelong vitality
sources   balanced   outsmarted   achieved

I have been helping women to outsmart their female fatigue for almost twenty years, and I've witnessed thousands of liberating transformations from exhaustion to enlightenment—when women have said "Enough is enough!" and taken charge to recharge their energy and revitalize their lives. Here are a few of the powerful words my clients have used to describe their energy transformations:

- "I keep my chin up, look life straight in the eye, and decide what's worth my time and what isn't."
- "I've finally realized that there isn't a prize for the weariest woman in the world, so why bother pushing myself so hard?"
- "When fatigue hits, instead of saying 'Oh no, I'm tired. I have to fight it and move on,' I now say, 'Okay, I'm tired. What is my body trying to tell me?' "
- "When I started saying 'no' to draining obligations, I started saying 'yes' to taking care of myself."
- "I used to think about adding more to my day—now my goal is to do less."
- "I ask for help when I'm feeling overwhelmed—and it feels great!"
- "Instead of thinking that I don't have the time to take care of myself, I now realize that I can't afford not to."
- "My goal in life is no longer to accomplish my to-do list—it's to live each day to its fullest."
- "When I'm tired, I rest. It's that simple."
- "I used to go, go, go. And I still go, but at least I stop every now and then to rest."
- "It finally dawned on me that I'm the only one responsible for my destiny."

How would you describe your energy transformation? Whether you have one of your own or identify with one of the above, use it as your life motto and remind yourself of it every day.

You Must Remember This

If you're anything like me, you've forgotten much of what you read in the last paragraph, never mind the first page of this book. When the hectic pace of life gets the better of you, keep these five important female facts in mind to keep you on track in outsmarting your female fatigue and mastering your female power:

1. When you *feel* tired, accept the fact that you *are* tired.

2. Your hormones, brain chemicals, blood sugar levels, connected brain, and biological rhythms keep you in close communication with your body's fatigue level—telling you when it's time to rest, refuel, and replenish with one or more of the 8 natural energy sources.

3. You may "feel" fatigue more than a man, but you can also feel more alive and energetic when you take the time to replenish your body. You have the potential to feel twice as energized by exercise, five times as energized by food, and ten times as energized by touch.

4. Your fatigue is not telling you that you aren't good enough, orga- nized enough, productive enough, or disciplined enough. But it may be telling you that you aren't eating enough, drinking enough, moving enough, sleeping enough, socializing enough, laughing enough, or relaxing enough.

5. Fatigue is a warning sign from your body that your energy equation is out of balance—and when you heed that warning and use your energy crisis positively, you'll recapture the essence of your life today and always.

You may be on the last page of this book, but the benefits of out-smarting your female fatigue will last the rest of your life.

THE TWENTY-FIRST—CENTURY WOMAN:
FROM TIRED TO INSPIRED

As we enter this new millennium, let's all join forces to make the female energy crisis an aberration of the twentieth century—a temporary loss of vitality that women quickly solved and turned around by proving to themselves and society that they had the smarts, savvy, and intellect to prioritize their life choices—and restore themselves physically, emotionally, spiritually, and nutritionally.

We can do it! Women comprise 52 percent of the population. We are the majority, and our ability to change is amazing. We've changed the world in many ways over the last century; now it's time to change ourselves in this new century—to redirect our attention inward to nurturing our bodies, recharging our energy, and reclaiming our vitality.

So start spreading the word to women across the globe. Help your daughters, granddaughters, nieces, sisters, coworkers, and friends feel empowered by life instead of exhausted by it. Share the 8 energizing strategies, offer insight to the fatigued women in your community, and be living proof of how the female energy crisis can be solved naturally, simply, and permanently. You'll not only brighten the vitality in your own life, but also in the world around you.

Additional Resources

EATING JOURNALS AND OTHER PUBLICATIONS

For journals, workbooks, articles, and other materials helpful in changing lifestyle habits, enhancing body image, and boosting self-esteem, visit our website at **waterhousepublications.com** or write to:

> Waterhouse Publications
> P.O. Box 4735
> Portland, ME 04112

SEMINARS AND WORKSHOPS

If your organization is interested in a presentation on *Outsmarting Female Fatigue* or other women's health topics, please contact:

> Debra Waterhouse
> PMB 342
> 6114 LaSalle Avenue
> Oakland, CA 94611

Bibliography

BOOKS

Albert, K.A. *Get a Good Night's Sleep*. New York: Fireside Books, 1996.

Andes, K. *A Woman's Book of Strength*. New York: Perigee, 1995.

Atkinson, H. *Women and Fatigue*. New York: Pocket Books, 1985.

Bailey, C. *Smart Exercise*. New York: Houghton Mifflin, 1994.

Bailey, C., and L. Bishop. *The Fit or Fat Woman*. Boston, MA: Houghton Mifflin, 1989.

Ball, N., and N. Hough. *The Sleep Solution*. Berkeley, CA: Ulysses Press, 1998.

Bell, D.S. *Curing Fatigue*. Emmaus, PA: Rodale Press, 1993.

Benson, H. *The Relaxation Response*. New York: Avon Books, 1975.

———. *Timeless Healing*. New York: Scribner, 1996.

Berdanier, C.D. *Advanced Nutrition: Micronutrients*. Boca Raton, FL: CRC Press, 1998.

Berne, K. *Running on Empty*. Alameda, CA: Hunter House, 1992.

Berry, C.R. *Is Your Body Trying to Tell You Something?* Berkeley, CA: Page Mill Press, 1997.

Birch, B.B. *Power Yoga*. New York: Simon & Schuster, 1995.

Blair, S.N. *Living with Exercise*. Dallas, TX: American Health Publishing, 1991.

Bogert, L.J. *Diet and Personality*. Garden City, NY: Garden City Publishing, 1934.

Borysenko, J. *Minding the Body, Mending the Mind*. New York: Bantam Books, 1987.

———. *A Woman's Book of Life*. New York: Riverhead Books, 1996.

Campbell, A. *The Sense of Well Being in America*. New York: McGraw-Hill, 1981.

Christie, C., and S. Mitchell. *Smart Cookies Don't Get Stale*. New York: Kensington Books, 1999.

Collinge, W. *Recovering from Chronic Fatigue: A Guide to Self-Empowerment*. New York: Perigee, 1993.

Cousins, N. *Anatomy of an Illness*. New York: W.W. Norton, 1979.

Davis, E. *Women, Sex, and Desire*. Alameda, CA: Hunter House, 1995.

Dement, W.C., and C. Vaughan. *The Promise of Sleep*. New York: Delacorte Press, 1999.

Dixon, M. *Love the Body You Were Born With*. New York: Perigee, 1996.

Donoghue, P.J., and M.E. Siegel. *Sick and Tired of Feeling Sick and Tired*. New York: W.W. Norton, 1992.

Edell, D. *Eat, Drink, and Be Merry*. New York: HarperCollins, 1999.

Eden, D. *Energy Medicine*. New York: Tarcher/Putnam, 1998.

Fahey, T.D., and G. Hutchinson. *Weight Training for Women*. Mountain View, CA: Mayfield Publishing, 1992.

Fisher, E. *The First Sex*. New York: Random House, 1999.

Fraser, L. *Losing It: America's Obsession with Weight and the Industry That Feeds It*. New York: Dutton Books, 1997.

Goodman, W.C. *The Invisible Woman*. Carlsbad, CA: Gurze Books, 1995.

Graber, R. *How to Get a Good Night's Sleep*. Minneapolis, MN: Chronimed Publishing, 1995.

Gray, J. *Mars and Venus in the Bedroom*. New York: HarperCollins, 1995.

Green, B., and O. Winfrey. *Make the Connection*. New York: Hyperion, 1996.

Hirsch, A.R. *Scentsational Sex*. Boston: Element Books, 1998.

Hirschmann, J.R., and C.H. Munter. *Overcoming Overeating*. New York: Fawcett Columbine, 1988.

―――. *When Women Stop Hating Their Bodies*. New York: Fawcett Columbine, 1995.

Hochchild, A.R. *The Second Shift*. New York: Avon Books, 1989.

Horne, J. *Why We Sleep*. New York: Oxford University Press, 1988.

Howard, B. *Mind Your Body: A Sexual Health and Wellness Guide for Women*. New York: St Martin's Griffin, 1998.

Jackson, D. *How to Make the World a Better Place for Women*. New York: Hyperion, 1992.

Janus, S., and C. Janus. *The Janus Report on Sexual Behavior*. New York: John Wiley and Sons, 1994.

Johnson, C.A. *Self-Esteem Comes in All Sizes*. New York: Doubleday, 1995.

Johnston, J.E. *Appearance Obsession*. Deerfield Beach, FL: Health Communications, 1994.

Kabatznick, R. *The Zen of Eating*. New York: Perigee, 1998.

Kortge, C. *The Spirited Walker*. San Francisco: HarperCollins, 1998.

Lark, S.M. *Chronic Fatigue Self-Help Book*. Berkeley, CA: Celestial Arts, 1995.

Lavery, S. *The Healing Power of Sleep*. New York: Fireside Books, 1997.

Lee, V. *Quiet Places*. Pleasantville, NY: Reader's Digest, 1998.

Mahle, J., and L. Jaffee. *The Bodywise Woman*. Champaign, IL: Human Kinetics, 1996.

McGhee, P.E. *Health, Healing, and the Amuse System*. Dubuque, IA: Kendall/Hunt Publishing, 1996.

Mellin, L. *The Solution: Winning Ways to Permanent Weight Loss*. New York: Regan Books, 1997.

Michael, R. *Sex in America: A Definitive Survey*. New York: Warner Books, 1995.

Mitchell, S., and C. Christie. *I'd Kill for a Cookie: A Simple Six-Week Plan to Conquer Stress Eating*. New York: Dutton Books, 1997.

Nelson, M. *Strong Women Stay Young*. New York: Bantam Books, 1997.

Northrup, C. *Women's Bodies, Women's Wisdom*. New York: Bantam Books, 1998.

Orenstein, P. *Flux: Women on Sex, Work, Kids, Love, and Life in a Half-Changed World*. New York: Doubleday, 2000.

Ornish, D. *Love and Survival*. New York: HarperCollins, 1997.

Pearsall, P. *The Pleasure Principle*. Alameda, CA: Hunter House, 1996.

Peterson, J.C., C. Bryant, and S. Peterson. *Strength Training for Women*. Champaign, IL: Human Kinetics, 1995.

Reichman, J. *I'm Not in the Mood*. New York: William Morrow, 1998.

———. *I'm Too Young to Get Old*. New York: Times Books, 1996.

Rodin, J. *Body Traps*. New York: Quill, 1992.

Roizen, M.F. *Real Age*. New York: Cliff Street Books, 1999.

Rosenthal, N.E. *Winter Blues*. New York: Guilford Press, 1999.

Roth, G. *Appetites*. New York: Dutton Books, 1996.

———. *Breaking Free from Compulsive Overeating*. New York: Bobbs-Merrill, 1990.

———. *When Food Is Love*. New York: Plume Books, 1991.

————. *When You Eat at the Refrigerator, Pull Up a Chair*. New York: Hyperion, 1998.

Serure, P. *Three Days to Vitality*. New York: Cliff Street Books, 1997.

Siegel, B. *Love, Medicine, and Miracles*. New York: HarperCollins, 1990.

Somer, E. *Age-Proof Your Body*. New York: William Morrow, 1998.

————. *Food and Mood*. New York: Henry Holt and Co., 1995.

————. *Nutrition for Women*. New York: Henry Holt and Co., 1993.

Stacey, M. *Consumed: Why Americans Love, Hate, and Fear Food*. New York: Simon & Schuster, 1994.

Sweeney, J. *I Know I Should Exercise, But* . . . San Diego, CA: Pacific Valley Press, 1998.

Taylor, S. *Sexual Radiance*. New York: Harmony Books, 1998.

Thayer, R. *The Origin of Everyday Moods*. New York: Oxford University Press, 1996.

Tribole, E. *Stealth Health*. New York: Viking, 1999.

Tribole, E., and E. Resch. *Intuitive Eating*. New York: St. Martin's Press, 1995.

Tyler, V.E. *Herbs of Choice*. New York: Pharmaceutical Products Press, 1994.

Waterhouse, D. *Outsmarting the Midlife Fat Cell*. New York: Hyperion, 1998.

————. *Like Mother, Like Daughter*. New York: Hyperion, 1997.

————. *Why Women Need Chocolate*. New York: Hyperion, 1995.

————. *Outsmarting the Female Fat Cell*. New York: Warner Books, 1993.

Weil, A. *Eight Weeks to Optimal Healing*. New York: Knopf, 1997.

————. *Natural Health, Natural Medicine*. New York: Houghton Mifflin, 1995.

Wells, C.L. *Women, Sport, and Peformance*. Champaign, IL: Human Kinetic Publishers, 1985.

Witkin, G. *The Female Stress Syndrome*. New York: Newmarket Press, 1991.

Wright, A., S. Nissenberg, and B. Manis. *Foods to Stay Vibrant, Young, and Healthy*. Minneapolis, MN: Chronimed Publishing, 1995.

Zerbe, K.J. *The Body Betrayed*. Carlsbad, CA: Gurze Books, 1993.

ARTICLES

Adler, J. "Stress." *Newsweek*, June 14, 1999, p. 56.

Anderson, I.M., et al. "Dieting reduces plasma tryptophan and alters brain 5-HT function in women." *Psychological Medicine* (1990), vol. 20, p. 785.

Antinoro, L. "Need pep? Know your energy-boosting options and make them work for you." *Environmental Nutrition*, September 1999, p. 1.

Arciero, P.J., et al. "Resting metabolic rate is lower in women than in men." *Journal of Applied Physiology* (1993), vol. 75, p. 2514.

Atkinson, H. "Just the facts." *Living Fit*. November/December 1997, p. 22.

Barclay, C., et al. "Dependence of muscle fatigue on stimulation protocol: Effect of hypocaloric diet." *Journal of Applied Physiology* (1992), vol. 72, p. 2278.

Barlow, C.E., et al. "Physical fitness, mortality, and obesity." *International Journal of Obesity* (1995), vol. 9, p. S41.

Barr, S.I. "Energy intakes are higher during the luteal phase of ovulatory menstrual cycles." *American Journal of Clinical Nutrition* (1995), vol. 61, p. 39.

Barr, S.I., et al. "Restrained eating and ovulatory disturbances: Possible implications for bone health." *American Journal of Clinical Nutrition* (1994), vol. 59, p. 92.

Begley, S. "Gray matters." *Newsweek*, March 27, 1995, p. 48.

Beidleman, B.A., et al. "Energy balance in female distance runners." *American Journal of Clinical Nutrition* (1995), vol. 61, p. 303.

Bennett, C., et al. "Short-term effects of dietary fat ingestion on energy expenditure and nutrient balance." *American Journal of Clinical Nutrition* (1992), vol. 55, p. 1071.

Benton, D., et al. "Vitamin supplementation for one year improves mood." *Neuropsychobiology* (1995), vol. 32, p. 98.

Berkman, L.F. "The role of social relations in health promotion." *Psychosomatic Medicine* (1995), vol. 57, p. 245.

Bernardo, H.D., et al. "A residue of transition: Jobs, careers, and spouse's time in housework." *Journal of Marriage and the Family* (1987), vol. 49, p. 381.

Blair, S.N., et al. "Changes in physical fitness and all-cause mortality: A prospective study of healthy and unhealthy men." *Journal of the American Medical Association* (1995), vol. 273, p. 1093.

Blair, S.N., et al. "Physical fitness and all-cause mortality: A prospective study of healthy men and women." *Journal of the American Medical Association* (1989), vol. 262, p. 2395.

Blum, I., et al. "Food preferences, body weight, and platelet-poor plasma serotonin and catecholamines." *American Journal of Clinical Nutrition* (1993), vol. 57, p. 486.

Blundell, J.E. "Serotonin and the biology of feeding." *American Journal of Clinical Nutrition* (1992), vol. 55, p. 155S.

Bortz, W.M., et al. "Catecholamine, dopamine, and endorphin levels during extreme exercise." *New England Journal of Medicine* (1982), vol. 305, p. 466.

Bowen, S.A.A., et al. "Influences of eating patterns on change to a low-fat diet." *Journal of the American Dietetic Association* (1993), vol. 93, p. 1309.

Brody, L. "Dieting on the dark side." *Shape*, March 1997, p. 108.

———. "Mindful muscles." *Shape*, December 1998, p. 86.

———. "*Shape* 1999 body image survey results." *Shape*, June 1999, p. 150.

Brownell, K.D., et al. "Medical, metabolic, and physiological effects of weight cycling." *Archives of Internal Medicine* (1994), vol. 154, p. 1325.

Butler, R. "Quality of life: Can it be an endpoint? How is it measured?" *American Jounal of Clinical Nutrition* (1992), vol. 55, 1267.

"Caffeine: Not so bad for your bones after all." *Tufts University Diet and Nutrition Letter*, September 1997, p. 1.

"Calcium supplements alleviate PMS symptoms." *Women's Health Advocate*, October 1998, p. 7.

Calles-Escandon, J., et al. "Basal fat oxidation decreases with aging in women." *Journal of Applied Physiology* (1995), vol. 78, p. 266.

"Can green tea help prevent cancer?" *UC Berkeley Wellness Letter*, December 1997, p. 1.

Caputo, F.A., et al. "Human dietary responses to perceived manipulation of fat content in a midday meal." *International Journal of Obesity Related Metabolic Disorders* (1993), vol. 17, p. 237.

Clemens, L.H., et al. "The effect of eating out on quality of diet in premenopausal women." *Journal of the American Dietetic Association* (1999), vol. 99, p. 442.

Coffey, C.E., et al. "Sex differences in brain aging." *Archives of Neurology* (1998), vol. 55, p. 169.

Cogan, R., et al. "Effects of laughter and relaxation on discomfort thresholds." *Journal of Behavioral Medicine* (1987), vol. 10, p. 139.

Colino, S. "The best vitamins for women." *American Health*, January 1999, p. 91.

"Conversations with Joan Borysenko." *American Health*, July/August 1998, p. 29.

Costill, D.L., et al. "Carbohydrate nutrition and fatigue." *Sports Medicine* (1992), vol. 13, p. 86.

Dallongeville, J., et al. "Influence of alcohol consumption and various beverages on waist girth and waist-to-hip ratio in a sample of French men and women." *International Journal of Obesity* (1998), vol. 21, p. 1178.

"Dehydrating effects of caffeine overstated." *Tufts University Health and Nutrition Letter*, July 1998, p. 1.

Dittus, K., et al. "Benefits and barriers to fruit and vegetable intake: Relationship between attitudes and consumption." *Journal of Nutrition Education* (1995), vol. 27, p. 120.

"Doctors 'supplement' their income." *UC Berkeley Wellness Letter*, June 1999, p. 2.

Donahey, K., et al. "Gender differences in factors associated with hypoactive sexual desire." *Journal of Sex and Marital Therapy* (1993), vol. 19, p. 25.

Dorsey, C.M., et al. "Effects of passive body heating on the sleep of older female insomniacs." *Journal of Geriatric Psychiatry and Neurology* (1996), vol. 9, p. 83.

Driver, H., et al. "Sleep disturbances and exercise." *Sports Medicine* (1996), vol. 21, p. 1.

Eastman, C.I., et al. "Bright light treatment of winter depression." *Archives of General Psychiatry* (1998), vol. 55, p. 883.

Engels, H.J., et al. "No ergogenic effects of ginseng during graded maximal aerobic exercise." *Journal of the American Dietetic Association* (1997), vol. 97, p. 1110.

"Exercise may strengthen creative powers." *Tufts University Health and Nutrition Letter*, March 1998, p. 2.

Feunekes, G.I.J., et al. "Food choices and fat intakes of adolescents and adults: Associations of intakes within social networks." *Preventive Medicine* (1998), vol. 27, p. 645.

Fisher, B. "Successful aging, life satisfaction, and generativity in later years." *International Journal of Aging* (1995), vol. 41, p. 239.

Fraser, L. "Glamour survey results: Body love, body hate." *Glamour*, October 1998, p. 280.

Friedenreich, C.M., et al. "Epidemiologic issues related to the association between physical activity and breast cancer." *Cancer* (1998), vol. 83, p. 600.

Gallup Organization. "Gallup survey of public opinion regarding diet and health." Prepared for the American Dietetic Association. Princeton, NJ: Gallup Organization, 1990.

Gallup Organization. "Women's knowledge and behavior regarding health and fitness." Conducted for the American Dietetic Association and Weight Watchers. June 1993.

Gardner, A.W., et al. "Physical activity is a significant predictor of body density in women." *American Journal of Clinical Nutrition* (1993), vol. 57, p. 8.

George, M.S., et al. "Brain activity during transient sadness and happiness in healthy women." *American Journal of Psychiatry* (1995), vol. 152, p. 341.

"Ginseng: Many forms, many questions, not enough answers." *Environmental Nutrition*, June 1998, p. 8.

Glanz, K., et al. "Why Americans eat what they do: Taste, nutrition, convenience, and weight control concerns as influences on food consumption." *Journal of the American Dietetic Association* (1998), vol. 98, p. 1118.

Glatzer, R. "Living to 100." *American Health*, July 1997, p. 56.

Golay, A., et al. "Similar weight loss with low or high carbohydrate diets." *American Journal of Clinical Nutrition* (1996), vol. 63, p. 174.

Gold, P. "Role of glucose in regulating the brain and cognition." *American Journal of Clinical Nutrition* (1995), vol. 61, p. 987S.

Goldstein, D.J. "Beneficial health effects of modest weight loss." *International Journal of Obesity Related Metabolic Disorders* (1992), vol. 16, p. 397.

Gornall, J., et al. "Short-term changes in body composition and metabolism with severe dieting and resistance exercise." *International Journal of Sports Nutrition* (1996), vol. 6, p. 285.

Gower, T. "Take a Deep Breath." *Health*, January/February 1998, p. 88.

Grant, J.E., et al. "Analysis of dietary intake and selected nutrient concentrations in patients with chronic fatigue syndrome." *Journal of the American Dietetic Association* (1996), vol. 96, p. 383.

Green, J., et al. "The healing energy of love." *Alternative Therapies in Health and Medicine* (1996), vol. 2, p. 46.

Green, M., et al. "Impaired cognitive functioning during spontaneous dieting." *Psychological Medicine* (1995), vol. 25, p. 1003.

Hanes, P.S., et al. "Trends in breakfast consumption of U.S. adults between 1965 and 1991." *Journal of the American Dietetic Association* (1996), vol. 96, p. 464.

Helgeson, V.S., et al. "Social support and adjustment to cancer." *Health Psychology* (1996), vol. 15, p. 135.

Herbert, J. "Sexuality, stress, and the chemical architecture of the brain." *Annual Review of Sexual Research* (1996), vol. 7, p. 1.

Hess, M.A. "Taste: The neglected nutrition factor." *Journal of the American Dietetic Association* (1997), vol. 97, p. S205.

Hill, M.A. "Light, circadian rhythms, and mood disorders: A review." *Annals of Clinical Psychiatry* (1992), vol. 4, p. 131.

Hogan, M. "The naked truth." *Fitness*, January/February 1998, p. 116.

Howard, B. "Survey says: *Shape* readers on body image and sex." *Shape*, September 1997, p. 118.

Ironson, G.T., et al. "Massage therapy is associated with enhancement of the immune system's cytotoxic capacity." *International Journal of Neuroscience* (1996), vol. 84, p. 205.

"Is your sunscreen blocking out an important vitamin?" *Environmental Nutrition*, July 1995, p. 3.

Jacoby, S. "Great sex." *Modern Maturity*, September/October 1999, p. 41.

Jenkins, D., et al. "Nibbling versus gorging: Metabolic advantages of increased meal frequency." *New England Journal of Medicine* (1989), vol. 321, p. 929.

Judge, G. "Let there be light." *American Health*, November/December 1998, p. 64.

Kanarek, R. "Psychological effects of snacks and altered meal frequency." *British Journal of Nutrition* (1997), vol. 77, p. S105.

Karklin, A., et al. "Restricted energy intake affects noctural body temperature and sleep patterns." *American Journal of Clinical Nutrition* (1994), vol. 59, p. 346.

Keim, N.L., et al. "Body fat percentage and gender: Associations with energy expenditure, substrate utilization, and mechanical work efficiency." *International Journal of Sports Nutrition* (1996), vol. 6, p. 356.

Kelly, A.K. "You think, therefore you heal." *Shape*, March 1999, p. 90.

Kendler, K.S. "Social support: A genetic-epidemiological analysis." *American Journal of Psychology* (1997), vol. 154, p. 1398.

Kleiner, S.M. "Water: An essential but overlooked nutrient." *Journal of the American Dietetic Association* (1999), vol. 99, p. 200.

Klem, M.L., et al. "A descriptive study of individuals successful at long-term maintainence of substantial weight loss." *American Journal of Clinical Nutrition* (1997), vol. 66, p. 239.

Kretsch, M.J., et al. "Cognitive effects of a long-term weight reducing diet." *International Journal of Obesity* (1997), vol. 21, p. 14.

Kripke, D.F. "Light treatment for nonseasonal depression: Speed, efficacy and combined treatment." *Journal of Affective Disorders* (1998), vol. 49, p. 109.

Krtiz-Silverstein, D., et al. "Employment status and heart disease risk factors in middle-aged women: The Rancho Bernardo study." *American Journal of Public Health* (1992), vol. 82, p. 215.

La Rue, A., et al. "Nutritional status and cognitive functioning in a normally aging sample: A 6-year assessment." *American Journal of Clinical Nutrition* (1997), vol. 65, p. 20.

Labbott, S.M., et al. "The physical and psychological effects of the expression and inhibition of emotion." *Behavioral Medicine* (1990), vol. 16, p. 182.

Lahmann, P.H., et al. "Attitudes about health and nutrition are more indicative of dietary quality in 50- to 75-year-old women than weight and appearance concerns." *Journal of the American Dietetic Association* (1999), vol. 99, p. 475.

Landau, M.D. "The new healing hospitals." *American Health*, June 1999, p. 22.

Leibel, R.L., et al. "Changes in energy expenditure resulting from altered body weight." *New England Journal of Medicine* (1995), vol. 332, p. 621.

Lewis, C., et al. "Nutrient intakes and body weights of persons consuming high and moderate levels of added sugars." *Journal of the American Dietetic Association* (1992), vol. 92, p. 708.

Ljungdahl, L. "Laugh if this is a joke." *Journal of the American Medical Association* (1989), vol. 261, p. 558.

Lloyd, H., et al. "Acute effects on mood and cognitive performance of breakfasts differing in fat and carbohydrate content." *Appetite* (1996), vol. 27, p. 151.

"Low fat, low mood." *Eating Disorders Review*, May/June 1998, p. 5.

Martin, R.A., et al. "Sense of humor as a moderator of the relation between stressors and moods." *Journal of Personality and Social Psychology* (1983), vol. 18, p. 93.

Maughan, R.J., et al. "Recovery from prolonged exercise: Restoration of water and electrolyte balance." *Journal of Sports Science* (1997), vol. 15, p. 297.

Maunsell, E. "Social support and survival among women with breast cancer." *Cancer* (1995), vol. 76, p. 631.

Melanson, K. "Fat oxidation in response to four graded energy challanges in younger and older women." *American Journal of Clinical Nutrition* (1997), vol. 66, p. 860.

Meston, C. "Aging and sexuality." *The Western Journal of Medicine* (1997), vol. 167, p. 285.

"The missing dietary guideline: Enjoy your food." *Tufts University Health and Nutrition Letter*, July 1998, p. 3.

Model, S. "Housework by husbands: Determinants and implications." *Journal of Family Issues* (1981), vol. 2, p. 225.

"More Evidence for Exercise." *Harvard Woman's Health Watch*. March 1997, p. 1.

Murray, L. "Bedroom healing." *Longevity*, December 1994, p. 28.

Musselman, D.L., et al. "The relationship of depression to cardiovascular disease." *Archives of General Psychiatry* (1998), vol. 55, p. 580.

Nehlsen-Cannarella, S.L. "The effects of moderate exercise training on the immune system." *Medicine and Science in Sports and Exercise* (1991), vol. 23, p. 64.

Neuhauser-Berthold, M., et al. "Coffee consumption and total body water homeostasis as measured by fluid balance and bioelectrical impedance analysis." *Annals of Nutrition Metabolism* (1997), vol. 41, p. 29.

Newsholme, E.A., et al. "Physical and mental fatigue: Metabolic mechanisms and importance of plasma amino acids." *British Medical Bulletin* (1992), vol. 48, p. 477.

Norris, R. "When the vacation's over." *Shape*, April 1998, p. 30.

Oliwenstein, L. "When stress makes you fat." *Shape*, December 1998, p. 71.

Owens, J., et al. "Can physical activity mitigate the effects of aging in middle-aged women?" *Circulation* (1992), vol. 85, p. 1265.

Pariser, S.F., et al. "Sex and the mature woman." *Journal of Women's Health* (1998), vol. 7, p. 849.

Patterson, B. "Fruit and vegetables in the American diet: Data from the HANES II survey." *American Journal of Public Health* (1990), vol. 85, p. 236.

Pizziol, A. "Effects of caffeine on glucose tolerance: A placebo-controlled study." *European Journal of Clinical Nutrition* (1998), vol. 52, p. 486.

Poehlman, E., et al. "Determinants of decline in resting metabolic rate in aging females." *American Journal of Physiology* (1993), vol. 264, p. E450.

Poehlman, E., et al. "Resistance training and energy balance." *International Journal of Sports Nutrition* (1998), vol. 8, p. 143.

Points, D. "Better sleep from A to Zzz . . ." *American Health*, September 1998, p. 100.

Polivy, J. "Psychological consequences of food restriction." *Journal of the American Dietetic Association* (1996), vol. 96, p. 589.

Poothullil, J.M. "Maintenance of weight loss using taste and smell sensations." *Journal of Women's Health* (1999), vol. 8, p. 109.

Provine, R.R., et al. "Laughing, smiling, and talking: Relation to sleeping and social context in humans." *Ethology* (1989), vol. 83, p. 295.

Rao, L. "Weight loss news: Stop cravings with sunshine." *Prevention*, February 1999, p. 51.

Riggs, K., et al. "Relations of vitamin B_{12}, vitamin B_6, folate and homocysteine to cognitive performance in the Normative Aging Study." *American Journal of Clinical Nutrition* (1996), vol. 63, p. 306.

Rippe, J., et al. "Improved psychological well-being, quality of life and health practices in moderately overweight women participating in a 12-week structured weight loss program." *Obesity Research* (1998), vol. 6, p. 208.

Rippe, J., et al. "The role of physical activity in the prevention and management of obesity." *Journal of the American Dietetic Association* (1998), vol. 98, p. S31.

Rogers, P.J., et al. "Dieting, dietary restraint, and cognitive performance." *British Journal of Clinical Psychology* (1993), vol. 32, p. 113.

Rosen, R., et al. "Prevalence of sexual dysfunction in women: Results of a survey study of 329 women in an outpatient gynecological clinic." *Journal of Sex and Marital Therapy* (1993), vol. 19, p. 171.

Roust, L.R., et al. "Effects of isoenergetic, low-fat diets on energy metabolism in lean and obese women." *American Journal of Clinical Nutrition* (1994), vol. 60, p. 470.

Saab, P.G., et al. "Premenopausal and postmenopausal women differ in their cardiovascular and neuroendocrine responses to stress." *Psychophysiology* (1989), vol. 26, p. 270.

Santiago, N.M. "Shopping turns us on." *Living Fit*, May 1998, p. 21.

Sato, Y., et al. "Effects of long-term psychological stress on sexual behavior and brain catecholamine levels." *Journal of Andrology* (1996), vol. 17, p. 83.

Schlosberg, S. "A fast burn." *Living Fit*, November/December 1997, p. 106.

Schoeller, D. "Balancing energy expenditure and body weight." *American Journal of Clinical Nutrition* (1998), vol. 68, p. 956S.

Schwartz, M.W., et al. "The new biology of body weight regulation." *Journal of the American Dietetic Association* (1997), vol. 97, p. 54.

"Secret revealed: Big eaters who don't gain." *Prevention*, May 1999, p. 69.

"The secret to longevity." *Women's Health Advisor*, June 1999, p. 1.

Seidell, J.C., et al. "Overweight, underweight, and mortality: A prospective study of 48,287 men and women." *Archives of Internal Medicine* (1996), vol. 156, p. 958.

Serdula, M.K., et al. "Fruit and vegetable intake among adults in 16 states: Results of a brief telephone survey." *American Journal of Public Health* (1995), vol. 85, p. 236.

"Sexual dysfunction." *Harvard Women's Health Watch*, April 1999, p. 1.

Sharp, D. "Give your metabolism a lift." *Health*, March 1998, p. 32.

Shide, D.J., et al. "Information about the fat content of preloads influences energy intake in healthy women." *Journal of the American Dietetic Association* (1995), vol. 95, p. 993.

Smith, A. "Influences of meal size on post-lunch changes in performance efficiency, mood, and cardiovascular function." *Appetite* (1991), vol. 16, p. 85.

Smith, A., et al. "Effects of breakfast and caffeine on cognitive performance, mood, and cardiovascular functioning." *Appetite* (1994), vol. 22,
p. 39.

Smith, A., et al. "The influence of meal composition on post-lunch
changes in performance efficiency and mood." *Appetite* (1988), vol.
10, p. 195.

Smith, W.P., et al. "Meditation as an adjunct to a happiness enhancement
program." *Journal of Clinical Psychology* (1995), vol. 51, p. 269.

"Smoothies: Smash hits." *UC Berkeley Wellness Letter*, March 1999, p. 3.

Snyder, A.C. "Overtraining and glycogen depletion hypothesis." *Medicine
and Science in Sports and Exercise* (1998), vol. 30, p. 1146.

"Some supplements don't dissolve." *Tufts University Health and Nutrition
Letter*, November 1997, p. 1.

Somer, E. "The power of vitality." *Shape*, September 1998, p. 128.

————. "Sex boosters." *Shape*, February 1995, p. 91.

Stanton, J.L., et al. "2001: A food odyssey." *Food and Nutrition News*
(1990), vol. 62, p. 29.

"Stop, look, and lose." *Prevention*, August 1999, p. 61.

"Toss and turn together." *Consumer Reports on Health*, December 1994, p.
142.

Trudeau, E., et al. "Demographic and psychosocial predictors of fruit and
vegetable intakes differ: Implications for dietary interventions." *Journal
of the American Dietetic Association* (1998), vol. 98, p. 1412.

Tucker, D.M., et al. "Nutrition status and brain function." *American Journal
of Clinical Nutrition* (1990), vol. 52, p. 93.

Vallerand,R., et al. "Motivation in later life: Theory and assessment." *International Journal of Aging* (1995), vol. 41, p. 221.

Van Etten, L.K., et al. "Effect of an 18 week weight-training program on
energy expenditure and physical activity." *Journal of Applied Physiology*
(1997), vol. 82, p. 298.

"Vital statistics." *Health*, April 1998, p. 16.

"Vitamin D: Sunlight redeemed? Reducing osteoporosis and cancer risk."
Women's Health Advocate, February 1998, p. 1.

Wallace, J., et al. "Twelve-month adherence of adults who joined a fitness
program with a spouse versus without a spouse." *Journal of Sports
Medicine* (1995), vol. 35, p. 206.

Welland, D. "Brain boosters: Can supplements sharpen your memory?" *Environmental Nutrition*, October 1998, p. 1.

"We're not like men." *Harvard Women's Health Watch*, October 1994, p. 6.

"What we do when we skip lunch." *Health*, September 1997, p. 38.

"Why an aperitif is an appetizer." *Harvard Women's Health Watch*, April 1999, p. 7.

Wing, R., et al. "Cognitive effects of ketogenic weight-reducing diets." *International Journal of Obesity* (1995), vol. 19, p. 811.

Wolf, A.M., et al. "Women and alcohol: Nutritional concerns and consequences." *Nutrition and the M.D.*, December 1994, p. 1.

"Women get higher on the run." *Health*, March/April 1995, p. 11.

Wright, K.P., et al. "Caffeine and light effects on nighttime melatonin and temperature levels in sleep-deprived humans." *Brain Research* (1997), vol. 747, p. 78.

Wurtman, J. "Depression and weight gain: The serotonin connection." *Journal of Affective Disorders* (1993), vol. 29, p. 183.

Yovetich, N.A., et al. "Benefits of humor in reduction of threat-induced anxiety." *Psychological Reports* (1990), vol. 66, p. 51.

Zhu, Y.I., et al. "Iron depletion without anemia and physical performance in young women." *American Journal of Clinical Nutrition* (1997), vol. 66, p. 334.